# IT'S SIMPLE

# PHENOLIC COMPOUNDS HEAL

### Vibrant & Fragrant Foods

## LIDGEA CREERY MA

Creery, Lidgea
    It's Simple  Phenolic Compounds Heal
    ISBN- 13: 978-1984000866
    ISBN-10:  1984000861


Authors web page:

https://sites.google.com/site/authorlidgeacreery/



Publisher: Amazon Create Space

Printed in the United States of America


**Other Books by this Author**

**It's Simple:**
    Vitamins Heal
    Minerals Heal
    Phenolic Compounds Heal

# DEDICATION


To my dear father and mother,
Gerald and his happy little Jewel,
Who blessed me with life,
They are eternally loved by me.

# TABLE OF CONTENTS

# DISCLAIMER

The opinions expressed in this book are based upon my personal views and a reflection of my own ongoing investigation as connected to health, nutrition and disease. The information is not complete, nor does it cover all possible uses, benefits, diseases, actions, physical conditions, precautions, side effects, scientific research, or other possible conditions or treatments.

The information contained in this book is general in nature and for discussion purposes only. The information is made available with the understanding that the author and publisher are not engaged in rendering medical, health, psychological or any other kind of personal or professional advice or services. It does not provide health or medical advice, nor should it be relied upon in part or in its entirety as the foundation for any medical decision.

This information is not to be used for self-diagnosis or self-treatment. It is not to be used as a substitute for qualified, professional medical advice. One should always consult their physician and other competent medical and health professionals regarding health, nutrition, diet, disease, ailment, physical conditions and medical treatment.

No warranties or guarantees are implied or expressed by the author or publisher. The author or publisher disclaim all responsibility for any liability, for any loss or risk, whether it be personal or otherwise, which is a direct or indirect consequence incurred by the use of any of the information from this book.

Our position and rights are consistent: You are accountable for your own beliefs, inferences, choices, actions and consequences.

# INTRODUCTION

Does modern medicine have all the answers?

Haven't you ever wondered if modern drugs aren't really covering up the symptoms and not healing the real problem?

I believe that at times this may be the case.  Then again, they do have quick fixes for many health problems.  But are they really good for our bodies? All those side-effects?

What's the alternative if we don't use these modern pharmaceutical cures?

Is there any other choice?

In some cases, I believe so, especially in prevention.

Is what is written in this book QUICK FIXES to medical problems?

No.  I don't claim to have any quick fixes.

Some people want guarantees.  This book doesn't have any.  It just shows you what research studies claim.  I do not claim anything to be a cure, that's up to the medical profession.

Foods containing phenolic compounds don't usually work rapidly.  But sill, I encourage one to eat homegrown organic fruits and vegetables which might have more vitamins, minerals and phenolic compounds than mass produced grocery store produce.  By creating a healthier eating lifestyle, one might experience better health in time.  By the way, juicing fruits and vegetables seems to get good results.

With organically grown, phenolic compound-rich foods and herbs, it's still a natural process in which what may help one person, yet might not work for another.  All one can say is there seems to be a lot of research and truth out there that seems to show that there our food choices definitely affect our health and the possibility of having disease.

In this book, in "Possible Uses", some information is based in research and facts, as well as, alternative, traditional or folk lore remedies.  When there are no scientific research found, you will note, no footnote numbers next to these items.  But another twist is some scientific research will investigate folk lore remedies.  Those, I have given footnotes.  Where there are no footnotes listed, they might be used in alternative medicines, traditional medicines or as folk lore remedies.  If pharmaceutical companies can't patient it and make money off of it, they aren't going to research it.  Right?

Just like modern medicines, sometimes alternative remedies work, sometimes they don't, and sometimes they may work for one person but not for another and they too, may have some undesirable side effects, especially if used with incompatible drugs or nutrients.

But as for the author, I am willing to look at alternative uses for phenolic compounds, even folk lore remedies. Maybe the old-timers knew more about foods and herbs than modern people do.  Maybe they've seen certain foods work before and that's why the remedies have been passed down through generations.

I share this information with you, not stating that it is absolute truth but only that it might contain truth.  I have tried to share with you, the reader, some of the warnings and hope that you will do your own research, and as always, it is at all times best to seek out the care of your physician to advise you.

# How to Use this Resource!

In each segment of this book, I list several different areas of importance, which shall be discussed below.

**Possible Uses**

This section might disclose some possible physical/emotional/ mental health concerns for which the phenolic compound and related foods are used.

But some of these "Possible Uses" health issues used can be scientifically proven as beneficial, some make sense based on their properties, and some are based on folk lore, traditional use, unverified but may be useful, or maybe some may not even work at all, that's why I list it as "Possible Uses". This may serve as a possible resource in guiding you as you do your own research.

In the "Possible Use" area, I often use research to verify the possible health benefits for the phenolic compound. But sometimes the research isn't specific as to where the compound came from; how it was introduced into the body; whether it was tested on a human, animal, or in a petri dish or what the result of the testing was. As you can see, there are many variables. Please don't assume what the research is but seek out the truth for yourself, then consult with your physician. I do not profess having the answers. This is just a tool for you to explore the possibilities.

**Possible Benefits**

This section contains what possible effects the phenolic compound might have on the body. I found a variety of information among resources, so again, I list it as "Possible Benefits".

**Warnings, Precautions, and Side Effects**

Most of the natural food sources shouldn't cause any problems unless one has an allergy or uses in excess. Often the problems come in when one is using supplements or using the food as a drug and not just a food. It is always best to check with one's medical professional before changing one's diet or overloading a food product in an effort to use it as a drug.

I have not found all the warnings for this section, so my hope is that you will be careful, prudent and use the mineral in moderation, and do your own research. When trying a new food, one should always pay attention to how the food may affect oneself. And when one tries a new food, it's wise to not overdo it, and if there is a problem, to definitely, see your doctor.

**Food Sources**

I did the best I can at finding food sources for each phenolic compound but I'm sure many have been left out, especially with herbs. I will be disclosing more about herbs later.

The asterisk symbol "*" in the "Food Sources" section means "Best of the Rest", otherwise, more nutritious foods or ones with a higher phenolic compound concentration.

**Research**

I have tried to find some research to show you how the phenolic compound may affect you. I didn't usually research the simple things like allergies, digestion, headaches, skin problems, or stomach aches. But instead, I tried to focus on the more serious ailments like cancer, diabetes, heart disease, neurological disorders or radiation poisoning.

# PHENOLIC COMPOUNDS

## Flavonoids      Polyphenols

- Not a true vitamin.
- Good source of antioxidants.
- Enhances absorption and protection of vitamin C.
- Body can't make it and must come from the diet.
- 7 groups: flavonones, flavanols, flavones, flavonols, flavanonols, and isoflavones.
- Contains over 8000 falconoids[1], 4000 polyphenolic compounds, and 500 anthocyanin structures[2], of which I will explore a few.

Phenolic compounds are a class of chemical compounds consisting of hydroxyl-group (-OH) which is directly bonded to aromatic hydrocarbon and is known as phenols . Although they can be synthesized industrially, many believe the natural-ocurring compounds found in plants are more desirable.  They are closely associated with the sensory and nutritional quality of foods and are often used as flavoring or perfumes because of their pleasant odor.

Natural phenolic compounds from medicinal herbs and dietary foods have proved to be a very crucial function for prevention and treatment of cancer and other diseases. They might have  anti-inflammatory, anti-mutagenic,  antioxidant activity,  apoptosis by arresting cell cycle, chemopreventive properties, DNA binding inhibitor, the blocking of signal pathways, and so much more.

# Natural Monophenols

## Different Types of Natural Monophenols
- Apiole, carnosol, carvacrol, dillapiole, rosemarinol


## Apiole

### Possible Uses
- Aging, Alzheimer's[3], amenorrhea, appetite stimulant[4], arthritis, chronic breast lactation[5], chronic fatigue[6], contusions, diarrhea, digestive stimulant[7], enlarged glands[8], gout, hypothalamus-pituitary axis[9], infertility, joint pain, menstruation, obesity, PMS, rash, swelling breasts[10], upset stomach, rheumatoid arthritis, urinary tract infection, wrinkles

### Properties
- Abortifacient, anti-inflammatory, antifungal, antimicrocial, antinociceptive, antiproliferative, cercaricidal, diuretic, irritant, phototoxic

### Warning, Precaution, and Side Effects
- Do not use if pregnant.
- Concentrated use of celery can cause hepatosis, fatty liver, emaciatin, extensive mucosal bleeding, inflammatory haemorrhagic infiltration and problems in the gastrointestinal tract[11].
- Do not abuse, may cause fatal poisoning.

### Food Sources

- Almond, anise, beef, black pepper, Brazillian fungus Paracoccidioides resiliencies, California bay laurel, carrot, celery and seeds, cheese, cloves, cocoa/chocolate, cow milk, dill, lemon, mace, nutmeg, orange, parsley and seeds, peas, sassafras, soybean, tomato, walnut

## Carnosol

- Often paired with Rosmanol.

## Possible Uses

- Adenoma prevention[12], Alzheimer's[13], Apc-associated intestinal tumor genesis prevention[14], acute lymphoblast leukemia (ALL)[15], amyotrophic lateral sclerosis (ALS-Lou Gherig disease)[16], atherosclerosis[17], breast cancer[18], cell cycle modulation and apoptosis, colon cancer[19], gram (+ -) inhibitor[20], Huntington's[21], leukemia[22], liver cancer[23], lung cancer[24], memory (cholinergic)[25], Parkinson's[26], prostate cancer (Mediterranean Diet)[27], skin cancer[28], skin problems, skin whitening[29]

## Possible Benefits

- DNA fragmentation is slowed down[30]
- Restrains SNP-mediated glial cell death[31]

## Properties

- Anti-inflammatory[32], anticancer[33], antimicrobial, antioxidant, apoptotic[34], antitumor, chemopreventive, cytotoxic[35], DNA damage repair[36], lipid peroxidation inhibitors[37], neuroprotective, peroxyl radical (CCI3O2) scavengers[38], pro-apoptotic[39]

## Food Sources

- *Rosemary, sage

# Carvacrol

## Possible Uses
- Alzheimer's[40], Bacillus cereus[41], Bacillus bronchispti[42], Bacillus cereus[43], breast cancer, COX-2[44], candida albicans[45], coronary heart disease[46], E coli[47], fatty acid oxidation, liver cancer[48], mouth bacterial infections[49], non-small cell lung cancer[50], prostate cancer[51], Pseudomonas aeruginosa[52], salmonella, small-cell lung cancer, Staphylococcus aureus[53], yeast infections

## Possible Benefits
- Circulatory homeostasis[54]

## Properties
- AChe inhibitor[55], analgesic, angiogenic, anti-elastase, anti-inflammatory, antibacterial[56], anticancer, anticandidal, antifungal, antigenotoxic[57], antihepatotoxic, antimicrobial, antioxidant, antiparasitic[58], antiplaque, antiplatelet[59], antiproliferative, antispasmodic[60], antitumor[61], fungicide, hepatoprotective[62], herbicide, insecticidal, surface cleasing agent

## Warning
- Some wild oregano has been genetically engineered by injecting the stalks with noxious bacterial protein to increase carvacrol levels.

## Food Sources
- Dittany of Crete, marjoram, *oil of oregano, *oregano, pepperwort, pine (bark, needles, resin), savory, thyme, wild bergamot, *wild oregano oil

# Dillapiole

## Possible Uses
- Alzheimer's[63], Aspergillus flavus[64], Aspergillus niger[65], asthma, Bacillus cereus[66], bad breath, blood sugar control, breast cancer[67], candida albicans[68], cardiovascular[69], cholesterol control, colic, colon cancer[70], diabetes, diarrhea, E-coli[71], Enterococcus faecalis[72], eye problems, gas, gastrointestinal disorders, heartburn, Heliobacter pylori, insecticide, insomnia, lactation stimulant, liver cancer[73], malaria[74], menstral pain and problems, Penicillium islandicum[75], preservative, Pseudomanas aeruginosa[76], Saccaromyces cerevisiae[77], Salmonella choleraesuis[78], spermicide, Staphylococcus aureus[79], stomachache, Yersinia enterocolitica[80]

## Properties
- Anti-inflammatory, antibacterial, anticancer[81], anticonvulsion, antidiabetic, antifungal, antihouseflies, antihypercholesterolaemic[82], antihyperlipidaemic[83], antileishmanial[84], antimalarial[85], antimicrobial, antimycobactetial[86], antioxidant, antiseptic, antispasmodic, antitumor[87], antiulcer[88], antiviral, carminative, diuretic, galactagogue[89], insecticide

## Warning
- Do not use while pregnant or breastfeeding.
- In large doses, may cause drowsiness, light sensitivity, problems breathing, rash, swelling throat, vomiting..

## Food Sources
- Acassar Kernals (Brucea jawanica (L) merr.), apium nodiflorum, black caraway, bunium cylindricum, *dill, Indian dill, Malva aegyptiaca, perilla alliacea L., piper guineense, piper aduncum

# Rosemarinol

## Possible Uses
- Acute myeloid leukemia (AML)[90], Alzheimer's[91], cardiovascular, drug-resistant infections, mosquito deterrent (10% oil)[92], Lyme disease tick deterrent[93], Parkinson's[94], propionibacterium acnes

## Possible Benefits
- Natural food preservative.
- Long-chain polyunsaturated fat storage preservation.
- Acetylcholine transference.

## Properties
- Anti-inflammatory, antibacterial, antifungal, antimicrobial, boosts antioxidants, preservative

## Warning, Precautions and Side Effects
- Do not use if pregnant.
- Do not overuse, may be toxic.

## Food Sources
- Rosemary

# Anthocyanins

- Red, purple and blue pigment.
- pH in a stable low pH environment is at 8.0, the plant can become almost colorless but with an increase in acidity, it changes to a darker and darker color.

## Different Types of Anthocyanins:
- Cyanidin, delphinidin, malvidin, pelargonidin, peonidin, petunidin

## Possible Uses
- AIDS/HIV[95], Alzheimer's[96], amyotrophic lateral sclerosis (ALS - Lou Gherig)[97], blood circulation, blood clots, bruising, cardiovascular disorders[98], cataracts, colon cancer, diabetic retinopathy, diabetes (type 2)[99], diarrhea, dysentery, epilepsy, eye health, hemorrhoids, inflammation, hypertension, ischemia, liver disorders, macular degeneration[100], multiple sclerosis[101], neurodegenerative disorders[102], night blindness, osteoporosis, Parkinson's[103], pyrexia, spider veins, urinary tract infections, varicose veins, vascular diseases

## Possible Benefits
- Strengthens blood vessels.
- Decreases inflammation.
- Reduces cholesterol deposits in arteries and damage to artery walls.
- Able to cross the blood-brain barrier to prevent blood clots.
- Strongest benefits when all are used together, although cyanidin seems to have the strongest health benefits.

## Food Sources

- Black beans, black corn, black quinoa, black rice, blue corn, blue-flesh potatoes, legumes, pink corn, pink rice, pistachio nuts, purple broccoli, purple cauliflower, red beans, red broccoli, red cabbage, red carrots, red corn, red-flesh potatoes, red radishes, red rice, red onions, red sweet potatoes, root crops, tubers

## Cyanidin

- Red, orange, and blue pigments.
- Often used with malvidin.

**Possible Uses**
- Alzheimer's, autism spectrum, atherosclerosis, arthritis, blood pressure control, blood sugar control, candida parapsilosis, cancer, cardiovascular disease[104], cerebral ischemia[105], cholesterol control, colon cancer[106], diabetes[107], E coli[108], enterococcus faecalis[109], fatty liver disease[110], heart disease, ischemia reperfusion, leukemia[111], liver ischemia[112], lung cancer[113], myocardial ischemia[114], obesity[115], prostate cancer[116], short-term spatial memory[117], skin cancer[118], staphylococcus epidermidis[119], streptococcus mutans[120]

**Possible Benefits**
- Free radical-scavenger.
- Easily absorbed into plasma.
- Stronger than vitamins C, E, and reservation with antioxidant effects.
- Fights against mycotoxins.
- Reduces DNA fragmentation.
- Decreases proliferation of cancer cells.
- Increases endothelial nitric oxide synthase which hampers atherosclerosis thus thwarting heart disease and heart attacks.

## Properties
- Anti-inflammatory, anticancer, antimicrobial[121], antimutagenic, antioxidant, antitoxic (mycotoxins), cancer cell apoptosis, chemopreventive, diuretic, neuroprotective[122], vascular protective

## Food Sources
- Açai, apples, *berries, bayberry, bilberry, black bean, blackberry, black currant, black plum, black raspberry, *blackberry, blackcurrants, blue-berried honeysuckle, blueberry, cherry, *chokeberry, cranberry, *elderberry, grapes, hawthorn, hibiscus sabdariffa, loganberry, *Marion blackberry, mulberry, peach, pear, plum, pomegranate, red apple, red raspberry, sweet cherry, tart cherry, some nuts and vegetables

# Delphinidin

- Bluish red pigment.
- pH-sensitive, changes from blue to red with increased acidity.

## Possible Uses
- Alzheimer's[123], atherosclerosis[124], breast cancer[125], cancer, cardiovascular disease[126], colon cancer[127], coronary heart disease, diabetes, epilepsy, heart disease, liver fibrosis[128], neurodegenerative disease[129], obesity[130], Parkinson's[131], periodontitis[132], platelet thrombosis, prostate cancer[133], retinal disease[134], seizures[135], stroke[136], UV-induced skin problems[137]

## Possible Benefits
- Might preserve endothelium integrity.[138]

## Properties
   * Anti-angiogenic[139], anti-inflammatory, anticancer[140], antifibrotic[141], antioxidant, cytoprotective[142],  diuretic, neuroprotective[143]

## Food Sources
   * Bananas, bilberry, black beans, *blackcurrent, blueberry, Cabernet Sauvignon grapes, Concord grapes, cowpeas, cranberry, eggplant, hibiscus sabdariffa, pomegranate, strawberry tree fruit (Arbutus unedo), wild blueberry


## Malvidin

* Blue pigment
* Color of red wine.
* Slightly acidic.

## Possible Uses
   * Alzheimer's[144], breast cancer[145], cardiovascular disease[146], colon cancer[147], colorectal cancer[148], diabetes[149], diabetes eye health[150], gastric adenocarcinoma[151], leukemia[152], liver cancer[153], neurodegenerative disease[154], obesity[155], Parkinson's[156], prostate cancer[157], UV-induced photoaging

## Properties
   * Anticancer, antioxidant, antiradical[158], apoptosis, cytotoxic, estrogenic, neuroprotective[159]

## Food Sources
   * Bilberry, black bean, black rice, blue potatoes, *blueberry, bog blueberries, Concord grapes, potatoes[160], Prunus mandshurica, red grape juice, red wine[161], Riceberry rice bran, Vitis viniferous, *wild blueberry

# Pelargonidin

- Dark red or purple pigment.

**Possible Uses**
- Alzheimer's[162], blood sugar control[163], breast cancer[164], cardiovascular[165], colon cancer[166], colorectal, diabetes[167], gastrointestinal digestion, hemi-Parkinson[168], hepatitis B virus associated hepatoma[169], human cancer cell lines HepG2 and LS174T[170], liver cancer[171], neurodegenerative disorders, obesity[172], ovarian cancer, streptozotocin-induced diabetic neuropathic hyperalgesia[173]

**Properties**
- Anti-inflammatory, anticancer, antioxidant, apoptotic, hepatoprotective[174], neuroprotective

**Food Sources**
- Black raspberry, chokecherries, lychee, pomegranate, red berries, *red radish, red raspberry, Saskatoon berries, small red bean, strawberry, sweet cherry, Vitis viniferous & rotundifolia grapes (muscadine)

# Peonidin

- Purplish red pigment.
- pH sensitive changes from red to blue with increased acidity.

**Possible Uses**

- Bacillus subtilis[175], breast cancer[176], cardiovascular disease[177], cognitive functions[178], colon cancer[179], diabetes, Enterococcus faecalis, Escherichia coli[180], Listeria monocytogenes[181], Lewis Lung carcinoma[182], lung cancer[183], metastatic breast cancer, motor functions[184], obesity[185], Salmonella typhimurium[186], Staphylococcus aureus[187]

## Properties

- Anti-inflammatory gene expression[188], antimicrobial[189], antioxidant, antiproliferative[190], apoptotic, gram-positive/negative bacteria inhibition, hypercholesterolemia, pro-apoptotic[191]

## Food Sources

- Açai, black rice, blueberry, cherries, cranberry, Eugenia jambolana Lam berry (Jamun), European cranberry[192], grapes, morning glories (blue flower), muscadine grape, peonies, plums, *raw cranberries, red grape, roses, wild blueberry
- Frozen blueberries loose peonidin.

## Petunidin

- Dark red or purple pigment.

## Possible Uses

- Breast cancer (non-tumorigenic)[193], cardiovascular disease[194], colon cancer (non-tumorigenic)[195], colorectal cancer[196], diabetes[197], eye strain[198], hepatitis B-associated hepatoma[199], liver cancer[200], obesity[201], prostate cancer[202]

## Properties

- Anticancer[203], antiproliferative[204], antioxidant, apoptototic[205], chemopreventive

**Food Sources**

- *Bilberry, black bean, black currant, blueberry, bog blueberry, Camellia sinensis Sunrouge red leaf tea[206], Camellia taliensis Sunrouge red leaf tea[207], Chinese changbai blueberry[208], Concord grapes, cowbeans, Jamun (Eugenia jambolana Lam) longanberry, meoru (vitis coignetiae pulliat), muscadine grape, purple tomato

# Isoflavones    Phytoestrogens

## Different Types of Isoflavones/Phytoestrogens
- Daidzein, genistein, glycitein

## Possible Uses
- Hormonal related conditions:
    - Anxiety, benign prostatic hypertrophy[209], breast cancer[210], cyclical mastalgia[211], depression, dysmenorrhoea, endometrial cancer[212], fluid retention, headaches, hot flashes, menopausal symptoms, mood swings, night sweats, osteoporosis[213], ovarian cancer[214], PMS, testicular cancer[215], uterine cancer[216]
  - Alzheimer's[217], atherosclerosis[218], arthritis[219], Buergers Disease, coronary artery spasm[220], Crohns disease[221], hypertension, large bowel cancer[222], inflammatory bowel disease[223], migraine headaches, myocardial infarction stroke[224], Reynaud's Syndrome, rheumatic diseases[225], ulcerated colitis[226], urinary incontinence

## Warning, Precautions and Side Effects
- Mimics the estrogen hormone.
- Pre-puberty children and infants don't need estrogen.
- Can help fight adult estrogenic hormonal problems.
- High intake of daidzein and genistein can have an undesirable effect on pituitary gland and thyroid function.[227]

## Food Sources
- Black cohosh, licorice root

# Daizein

## Possible Uses
- Alcohol addiction[228], allergies, Alzheimer's[229], atherosclerosis[230]bone density, bone formation and mass[231], breast cancer[232], cardiovascular disease[233], cervical cancer, cognitive function[234], colon cancer, dementia[235], diabetes (type 2)[236], endometrial cancer[237], hypertension[238], leukemia[239], menopausal symptoms[240], obesity (belly fat)[241], osteoporosis[242], postmenopause, prostate cancer[243] (+ fish)[244], stroke[245]

## Possible Benefits
- Helps protect cellular integrity.

## Properties
- Ameliorative[246], anabolic, anti-aging, anti-inflammatory, antiestrogenic, antioxidant, antiplatelet[247], antitumor[248],
- Estrogenic and anti-estrogenic.

## Warning, Precautions and Side Effects
- Can interfere with cancer drug Tamoxifen.
- Can cross the placenta.[249]
- Can be found in breast milk if mother eats isoflavones.
- Eat in moderation, might cause infertility or liver problems.

## Food Sources
- Alfalfa sprouts, chicpeas, fava beans, kudzu, legumes, lupine, meatless hotdogs/sausage, miso, peanuts, peas, psoralea,  red clover, soy-based infant formula, soybeans, soy products, soy protein isolates, tempeh, tofu

# Genistein

## Possible Uses
  • Alzheimer's[250], atherosclerosis[251], bladder cancer[252], bone density[253], breast cancer[254], cardiovascular disease[255], cervical cancer[256], cognitive function[257], colon cancer[258], dementia[259], diabetes[260], esophageal cancer[261], hypertension[262], lung cancer[263], obesity (visceral fat), ovarian cancer[264], Parkinson's[265], postmenopausal ailments[266], postmenopausal bone density[267], prostate cancer[268], stroke[269]

## Possible Benefits
  • Precursor legume antimicrobial effects.[270]
  • Helps with menopause and menstruation.
  • Blocks or regulates estrogen.

## Properties
  • Anthelmintic, anti-inflammatory[271], anticancer[272], antioxidant, chemoprotectant, immunomodulator[273], neuroprotective[274]

## Warning, Precautions and Side Effects
  • Crosses the placenta.[275]
  • Can be found in breast milk.[276]

## Food Sources
  • Alfalfa sprouts, barley, barley sprouts, broccoli, caraway, cauliflower, chicpeas, clover seeds, coffee, fava beans, *fermented soybean, flemingia vestita, kudzu, legumes, lupin, miso, soy-based infant formulas, *soybean, soy protein isolates, sunflower, tempeh, tofu

**Research**

Dietary flavonoids show protective properties in human ovarian cancer cells.  Six flavonoids: apigenin, genistein, kaempferol, luteolin, quercetin, and taxifolin were shown to inhibit cell growth. The inhibitory factors were genistein, kaempferol, apigenin, quercetin, as so on.  Genistein, quercetin, and luteolin have shown the strongest inhibition factors in human ovarian cancer cell proliferation.[277]

# Glycitein

**Possible Uses**

- Allergies, Alzheimer's, atherosclerosis[278], bone loss, breast cancer[279], cardiovascular disease[280], cervical cancer[281], colon cancer[282], colorectal cancer[283], diabetes (type 2)[284], endometrial cancer[285], endometriosis[286], heart disease, obesity[287], osteoporosis, ovarian cancer[288], Parkinson's, postmenopausal health, prostate cancer[289], stroke[290]

**Properties**

- Antioxidant, antiphotoaging, hypolipidemic[291], phytoestrogen

**Food Sources**

- Chic peas, *fermented soybeans, legumes, *soybean, soy protein isolates, tofu

# Phenolic Acid

## Different Types of Phenolic Acid
- Capsaicin, curcumin, ellagic acid, gallic acid, salicylic acid, tannic acid, and vanillin

## Possible Uses
- Atherosclerosis, cancer, HIV, haemophilus influenzae, ulcers

## Capsaicin

- Blood-thinner and pain-killer.

## Possible Uses
- AIDS/HIV[292], aches, acute thromboembolism[293], alcoholic tremors, Alzheimer's, arthritis[294], arthritis pain[295], bladder overactivity[296], blood pressure control[297], body warmer, bone cancer pain[298], bowel problems, burning foot syndrome, breast cancer[299], cancer, cardiovascular disease[300], chronic pain[301], chronic post herpetic neuralgia[302], circulation, cirrhosis circulation[303], cluster headaches[304], cold hands and feet, cold, colon cancer[305], congestion, cramps, delirium tremers, diabetic foot pain (Axsain), diabetic neuropathy[306], digestion, dispels mucus, dissolves blood clots, fibromyalgia[307], food nutrient absorption, foot warmer (Civil War), gastric ulcers[308], gout, HIV pain[309], headache, heart attack, heart tonic, herb catalyst, herpes simplex[310], herpes topical treatment[311], herpes zoster (shingles)[312], Hodgkins, hypertension circulation[313], IBS, joint problems, kidney stones, knee osteoarthritis, lung cancer[314], lupus, migraine, myocardial protective[315], nasopharyngeal[316], neuralgia, neurogenic inflammation[317], neuropathic pain[318], opens lung airways,

osteoarthritis[319], pancreatic cancer[320], Parkinson's, pleurisy, post-herpetic neuralgia (shingles)[321], prostate cancer[322], pruritus ani (rectum skin irritation), psoriasis, radiation, renal anxiety[323], renal colic[324], renal nausea[325], rheumatoid arthritis, shingles[326], shock, sinus headache[327], spasms, stimulates mucus release, stomach, stroke[328], surgical neuropathic pain[329], sweating promotion, toothache, uremic proritus[330], vasomotor rhinitis[331], weight loss
- Good for moderate use with long-standing chronic conditions.
- Leaves, stem, or fruit promote uterine contractions.

## Possible Benefits
- Pain reliever, boosts endorphins, often used topically.
- Clots blood internally and externally.
- Kills cancer.
- Aids with mineral absorption.
- Increases blood flow to skin (fever, sweating).
- Binds with cancer cell proteins in the mitochondria to trigger apoptosis of prostate cancer cells, or cell death without hurting healthy cells.
- Suppressed platelet aggregation better than aspirin and didn't affect blood coagulation.[332]
- Heat-activated receptor extracts burning pain to communicate information in central nervous system.[333]
- Important receptor for bone cancer pain, detects tissue acidosis.[334]

**Properties**

- Analgesic, anestetic, anti-inflammatory, antibacterial, anticancer, antihyperalgesic, antioxidant, antiproliferative[335], antiscorbutic, antiscrofulous, antispasmodic, antitumor, aperient, capsaicin pain blocker, cardiac tonic, carminative, coagulant, diaphoretic (breaks fever), diuretic, mutagenicity, neuroprotective[336], rubefacient, styptic, tumorigenicity, vasodialator, prevents blood platelets from bunching up and keeps it flowing, vulnerary

**Warning, Precautions, and Side Effects**

- FDA considers as generally safe.
- Do not use if pregnant or breastfeeding.
- Use in moderation.
- Tissue irritant.
- Often used topically.
- Burns if you get it into your eyes or open sores.
- Can be hot to the mouth, tongue and for some people, to the stomach.
- Applied to skin can trigger blisters, dilute first.
- Start with small dosages and build up.
- Some people may be allergic to it.
- Not good for acute inflammation.
- Do not use if you have asthma.
- Do not use if you have gastrointestinal problems, may cause ulcers.
- May hurt mouth, upset stomach, and give gastrointestinal pain.

- Overdose may cause gastroenteritis.
- Overdose may cause renal damage.
- Wash pepper off hands with vinegar but it's probably better to use gloves or put oil on hands before touching the pepper.
- May cause confusion, dizziness, fainting, heartburn, and weakness.
- Be careful when using it topically and frequently, as it may cause nerve damage.
- Might interact with ACE inhibitors, antihypertensive, MAO inhibitors, sedatives, and theophyllines.
- Severe exposure can cause death.
- Heat is measured by the Scoville heat scale.

**Note:  Milk and dairy products help temper the capsaicin oil, thus reducing the heat.**

**Counterirritants**
- Heet, Omega Oil, Milk, Stimurub

**Food Sources**
- Peppers -- the more capsaicin, the hotter the pepper.

**Research**

Capsaicin from hot chili peppers kill tumor cells.[337]

Research shows that capsaicin might be superior to aspirin and might prevent death by acute pulmonary thromboembolism.[338]

Dried Chili pepper (Capsicum Frutescens L.) extract showed results for cardiovascular disease to be better than acetosal in bleeding and clotting time.[339]

**Recipes**

**Cluster Headaches Remedy**
• Put capsaicin preparation of cayenne/water paste outside nose for 5 days, some people say to swab it inside nose, use your own judgment.  It's hot.
• Go and lay down for a while.
Warning: reports of burning nostrils and running nose.

**Cayenne Congestion Tea**
• Add a little ginger, horseradish or lemon
• 1/8-1/2 t. cayenne powder
• 1 c. hot water
• Dab of raw honey

**Shingles Topical Application**
• Over the counter creams, gels, liquids and ointments can be bought.
Warning: wear gloves to apply.

• Capsaicin treatment should be used for at least 4 weeks for substantial pain relief, with limited success. The more one uses it, the less burning one should feel.[340]

**Bleeding Wound Folk Treatment**
• Sprinkle a large amount of cayenne powder on wound, until it coagulates.

**Dr. Christoper's Heart Attack Tea**[341]
If conscious:
• Cayenne pepper has to be 90,000+ H.U.
• 1 t. powder in 1 c. warm water, drink
If unconscious
• Cayenne pepper has to be 90,000+ H.U.

- Cayenne tincture or extract
- A couple of full droppers, full strength, under tongue

I have great respect for Dr. Christoper and his knowledge of natural remedies. I received this information from an alternate source. See footnotes.

## Pepper Spray
- Use goggles, mask and rubber gloves to make.
- Hottest chili pepper you can find.
- Fine black pepper for coughing effect.
- Water and/or apple cider vinegar.
- Blend everything until very fine.
- Cook, screen then funnel into a spray bottle.

# Curcumin

## Possible Uses
- Alzheimer's[342], amyloidosis (fibril formation)[343], anterior uveitis[344], atherosclerosis[345], arthritis[346], atrial arrhythmias[347], breast cancer[348], cardiac hypertrophy[349], cardiovascular disease[350], chronic obstructive lung disease[351], chronic renal disease[352], Crohn's[353], colon cancer[354], diabetes[355], diabetic cardiovascular complications[356], familial adenomatous polyposis[357], fibromyalgia, gall bladder function, gastrointestinal symptoms, heart failure[358], hyper-cholesteremia[359], inflammatory bowel disease (IBD)[360], learning problems, leukemia, liver cirrhosis[361], liver disease (Hep3B)[362], lung cancer[363], lymphomas[364], memory problems, pancreatic cancer[365], pancreatitis[366], Parkinson's[367], prostate cancer[368], pulmonary disease[369], psoriasis[370], rheumatoid arthritis[371], stress, ulcerated colitis[372], ventricular arrhythmias[373]

## Possible Benefits

- Promotes cancer apoptosis.
- Lowers oxidative damage.
- Protects DNA pulmonary cells.
- Inhibits the formation of protein fragments in the brain.
- With Alzheimer's, it thwarts fibril and oligomer formation.
- Inhibits human blood platelet aggregation.

## Properties

- Angiogenesis inhibitor, anti-angiogenic, anti-inflammatory, anti-invasive[374], anticancer, anticarcinogenic[375], antioxidant, antiproliferative, antithrombotic[376], antitumor, catatonic, chemopreventive, chemoresistance[377], immunomodulator, immunosuppressive, radiosensitive (radiation-induced prosurvival gene)[378], radioresistance[379]

## Warning, Precautions, and Side Effects

- Low side effects.

## Food Sources

- Curry, *turmeric, yellow mustard

## Research

Three compounds arrested lung tumor formation. The nodules were inhibited by curcumin mostly, along with catechin, and lastly rutin.[380]

# Ellagic Acid

## Possible Uses
- Asthma[381], bladder cancer[382], breast cancer[383], cancer[384], cardiovascular[385], cholesterol control, Crohn's disease, colon cancer[386], esophagael cancer[387], female fertility[388], female offspring fertility[389], heart disease[390], liver damage, leukemia[391], lung tumorigenesis[392], men's reproductive health[393], osteoporosis[394], prostate cancer[395], respiratory system, small intestinal carcinomas[396], testicular health[397], UV-B skin wrinkles[398], ulcers

## Possible Benefits
- Helps maintain cellular homeostasis.
- Hampers pathogenic prokaryotes continued existence.
- Reduces platelet aggression.

## Properties
- Anti-aging, anti-inflammatory, anticancer, anticarcinogenic, antieosinophilic[399], antiestrogenic, antimutagenic[400], antioxidant (nuts), antiproliferative, apoptotic, chemopreventive, gastroprotective, nonspecific COX ingibitor

## Food Sources
- Almonds, apples, berries, black current, blackberries, cranberries, curcumin, false strawberry, grapes, nuts (antioxidant),*pomegranate, raspberry leaf[401], strawberries, thornless blackberry, tumeric, walnuts

# Gallic Acid

## Possible Uses
- AIDS/HIV, Alzheimer's[402], atherosclerosis[403], breast cancer[404], bronchitis, cancer, cardiovascular disease[405], colds, colon cancer[406], coughs, diabetes[407], leukemia[408], lung cancer[409], Parkinson's[410], prostate cancer[411], stroke[412]

## Properties
- Anti-inflammatory[413], anticancer[414], antileukemic[415], antimutagenic[416], antineoplastic, antioxidant[417], antiproliferative, antiseptic, apoptoxic, chemoprevention, hypolipidemic[418]

## Warning, Precautions, and Side Effects
Black, green, Oolong, and pu-erh tea have four catechins, caffeine and gallic acid.  Fermentaion lowers catechins, elevates gallic acid and lowers caffeine levels in Fujian Oolong.[419]

Tea also has fluoride which is greater in the non-organic teas.  Fluoride can cause bone calcification problems which will be discussed in volume 3 of this same series.

## Food Sources
- American oak, berries, blackberry, Boswellia dalzielii, clove, cocoa, golden root, grape seeds/skins, hot chocolate, hot cocoa, mango leaves and peel, Mediiterranean brown seaweed Cystoseira sedoides, milk chocolate, tea (black, green, Oolong, pu-erh), *piper betle L leaf extract (betelvine), plantago species, red raspberry, vinegar, walnut thin coating, wine, witch hazel

## Research

Piper betle L leaf extract has more lipid per oxidation prevention power than tea.[420]

## Salicylic Acid

### Possible Uses
• Acne, Alzheimer's oxidative damage detection[421], body aches and pain, breast cancer[422], COX-1[423], cardiovascular disease[424], colon cancer[425], colorectal cancer[426], coronary artery disease[427], diabetes (type 2)[428], flat facial warts[429], headaches, heart attack, heart failure[430], hypertension[431], leukemia[432], Parkinson's oxidative damage detection[433], recurrent pregnancy loss[434], stroke[435], wrinkles

### Possible Benefits
• Reduces blood platelet clotting.

### Properties
• Anti-inflammatory[436], antileukemia, antioxidant[437], antimicrobial[438], antiplatelet[439], antithrombotic, cardioprotective[440]

### Warning, Precautions and Side Effects
• Do not use if you have a blood clotting bleeding disorder.
• Do not use if you have bleeding ulcers.
• Aspirin allergies can include asthma.
• Heavy usage of aspirin, then stopping, might result in a blood clot.

### Food Sources
• Aspirin (acetyl salicylic acid), Gold Mohar, licorice, peanut, peppermint, wheat, willow leaves

# Tannic Acid

A specific form of tannin.
• Often used as a topical treatment.

## Possible Uses
• Blood pressure control[441], blood pressure drop with burn therapy[442], bloody urine, burn therapy (topical)[443], canker sores, childhood bronchial asthma[444], cold sores, colon cancer[445], coughs, diaper rash, dust mites[446], diarrhea[447], dysentery[448], fever blisters (topical)[449], flavoring agent, foot blisters, genital herpes (topical)[450], hemorrhoids, inflammatory bowel disease (IBD)[451], ingrown toenails, internal hemorrhoids[452], leather production[453], making ink, minor burns, oral herpes (topical)[454], osteoarthritis[455], painful joints, poison ivy, prickly heat, receding gums, skin rash, sore throat, sore tonsils, stop bleeding, sunburn, wood staining, wound treatment[456]

## Possible Benefits
• Tannic acid is used as a spray to get rid of dust mites and other indoor allergens to prevent allergies/asthma.
• Tannic acid and silver nitrate is often used together to treat wounds and burns.
• Constricts body tissue.

## Properties
• Anti-inflammatory, antifungal[457], antinociceptive, antioxidant, antitumor[458], antiviral[459], astringent, diuretic, pesticide

## Warning, Precautions and Side Effects
• Do not use if pregnant or breast feeding.
• Can cause gas and congestion.

- Do not use if you have kidney or liver problems.
- Do not bathe with tannic acid, especially if you have heart failure or infectious diseases.

**Food Sources**
- Black tea, grape seed extract, grape skin, green tea, oak trees, persimmons, Sicilian sumac leaves, spinacia oleracea leaves, witch hazel, unripe fruit

**Recipe**

**Universal Antidote for poisoning**
- Tannic acid
- Activated charcoal
- Magnesium oxide
Warning: Doesn't work.
- The problem is the charcoal inactivates the tannic acid.

**Tannic Acid Burn Treatment[460]**
- 2 T. dry powder
- 1 glass of water
- Makes a 2 1/2% mixture

**Leather Production Spray Solution[461]**
- Mimosa, querbracho or chestnut extract
- Hot water bark extract
- Prevents water loss in mucous membranes

# Tannins

- Polyphenolic compound has positive and negative attributes.

## Possible Uses
- Acne, arthritis, breast cancer[462], cancer protection[463], gastroduodenal disorders[464], HIV[465], helicobacter pylori[466], leukemia[467], prostate cancer[468], rheumatoid arthritis[469], Staphylococcus aureus[470], tans hides, UV-B radiation tumors[471], wood staining

## Possible Benefits
- Inhibited sister-chromatid exchanges and mutagenic bacterial chromosomal aberrations in DNA repair.[472]

## Properties
- Anti-inflammatory, antibacterial, antimicrobial, antioxidant, antiproliferation, astringent, cytotoxic[473], pesticide, skin protectant

## Warning, Precautions, and Side Effects
- Dry puckery feeling in mouth.
- Do not use if pregnant, may cause miscarriage, low birth weight and possibly other problems.
- Metal chelator: excessive usage of tannins inhibit mineral absorption, especially iron, copper, and zink, also may cause anemia.
- Avoid extreme use of tannin foods.
- May cause bowel irritation, headaches, kidney damage, liver damage, and stomach problems.
- Long term, high intake consumption is not recommended.
- Connection between esophageal or nasal cancer and regular consumption with high tannin herbs.

## Food Sources

- Most herbs and spices: cinnamon, cloves, cumin, tarragon, thyme, vanilla.
- Acacia, bayberry, berries, black tea, chestnut, chocolate, cleavers, coffee, comfrey, fruit juices, grape seed extract, grape skins, green tea, legumes, mangosteen fruit, nuts, peppermint, persimmons, pomegranates, sarsaparilla, silage, smoked foods, tea, unripe fruit, uva ursi, walnuts, wine yellow dock
- Red bean have highest and white beans have least in legumes.
- Sorghum is high in tannins.
- Most vegetation has tannins.

## Vanillin

- Catechol precursor.

## Possible Uses

- Acne, Alzheimer's[474], brain damage[475], breast cancer[476], cancer[477], cerebral ischemia[478], colorectal cancer[479], convulsive disorders[480], Cronobacter bacterial species[481], digestive problems, dizziness, epilepsy[482], headache, infantile convulsions[483], kidney, limb numbness[484], liver, Parkinson's[485], memory, prostate cancer[486], rheumatism[487], sickle-cell disease (vanillin derivative INN-312 & INN-298)[488], skin lightener, skin sensitizer, tetanus[489], vertigo[490]

## Possible Benefits

- Cronobacter bacterial can cross the blood brain barrier, thus causing enteritis and meningitis. Vanilla can be added to the food to thwart this bacteria.
- Inhibited mutagenic bacterial chromosomal aberrations in DNA repair.[491]

## Properties

- Anti-epileptic[492], anti-inflammatory, antibacterial, anticonvulsant[493], antimicrobial, antioxidant, antisickling[494], chemo preventive, hepatoprotective, neuroprotective[495], sedative[496]

## Food Sources

- Chinese red pine, cloves, fennel, Gastrodia elata blume[497], roasted coffee, Tianma Rhizoma Gastrodiae[498], vanilla beans

## Warning, Precautions and Side Effects

- Coffee has many negative side effects listed in the third book of this series.

## Recipe

### Homemade Vanilla Extract

- 8 long vanilla beans, split lengthwise down the middle
  - Different beans have different smells and flavor
- 8 oz. 35-40% food grade alcohol, organic grain alcohol, ethyl alcohol, Everclear, Vodka, Brandy, or Rum
- 10 oz. distilled water
- Put it into pint jar and place into cupboard for a couple of months, shake occasionally

# Flavan-3-ol

## Types of Flavan-3-ol
• Catechins, epicatechin, epigallocatechin, gallocatechin, theaflavin (reddish color in fermented tea), Theaflavin-3-gallate (black tea), Theaflavin-3,3'-digallate (black tea), thearubigins (tea during fermentation)

I will only be discussing the first three types.

## Warning, Precautions, and Side Effects
• Most of the research I found has been done on tea.  I don't list all the risks of drinking tea in this book but it will be found in further detail in the third book, "Healing Herbs" of this series.
I list tea because it can have health benefits if used prudently and wisely for medical reasons, not for using as a sweet water substitute.  It does have health risks.


## Catechins


## Possible Uses
• Age-related neurodegeneration[499], aging, Alzheimer's[500], arthritis[501], atherosclerosis[502], breast cancer[503], cancer chemoprevention[504], cancer  protection, cardiovascular disease, cholesterol control, dementia[505], diabetes[506], diabetes cataracts[507], diabetic blood sugar control (type 2)[508], dyslipidemia[509], fat reduction[510], HIV-associated neurocognitive disorder[511], hypercholesterolemia[512], hepatitis, influenza, ischemic cerebrovascular disease[513], ischemic heart disease[514], ischemic stroke[515], liver cancer[516], liver disorders[517], neurological disorders, neuropathic pain[518], non-

alcoholic fatty liver disease, obesity[519], Parkinson's[520], prostate cancer[521], stomach cancer[522], tumor formation, weight control,

## Possible Benefits
- Can cross the blood-brain barrier.
- Interacts with many human genes.
- Prevent blood vessel tumor growth.
- 2-6 hours after consuming cocoa, there were reductions in platelet primary hemostasis.
- 100 time stronger than the antioxidant vitamin C and 25 times more powerful than vitamin E.[523]
- (-)-Catechin represses Kruppel-like factor 7 expression.[524]

## Properties
- Anti-inflammatory, anti-influenza virus[525], antioxidant, anticancer, antidiabetic, antitumor, herbicide, histidine to histamine inhibitor, neuroprotective[526]

## Warning, Precautions and Side Effects
- Use with caution when pregnant, breastfeeding, elderly, skin problems or diabetic.
- Green tea might cause colon carcinogenesis.[527]

## Food Sources
- Acai oil, apple juice, apple peels, apricots, barley, black tea, blackberries, broad beans, buckwheat plant, cacao beans, cherries, chocolate, citrus, cocoa, cranberries, *dark chocolate, grape seed, grapes, *green tea (caffeine risks), lentils, nectarines, onions, peach, pears, plums (with skin), raisins, rhubarb, strawberry leaf (infection-inhibiting) tobacco, vinegar, white tea, wine
- In some bacteria and fungi.
- Some cacao products may have low bioavailability of catechins.[528]

# Epicatechin

## Possible Uses
- Alzheimer's[529], blood pressure reduction[530], breast cancer[531], cardiovascular disease[532], colon cancer[533], coronary atherosclerosis[534], diabetes (type 2)[535], HIV-associated neurological disorders[536], hepatitis C virus protection[537], insulin resistance, ischemic stroke, lung cancer[538], muscle fatigue, neurodegenerative,  obesity, pancreatic tumor[539], Parkinson's[540], prostate cancer[541], spatial memory[542], vascular protection[543]

## Possible Benefits
- Crosses the blood brain barrier.[544]
- Can increases testosterone secretion.[545]
- Inhibits platelet aggression and leukocyte migration.
- Platelet activity is reduced 2 hours after eating dark chocolate.[546]
- Dark chocolate eaten previous to a stroke can prevent some stroke damage.[547]
  - So you're justified in eating that dark chocolate candy bar.
- Aids with amyloid $\beta$ protein-induced apopsis[548],

## Properties
- Anti-inflammatory[549], anticancer, anticarcinogenic[550], antineurodegenerative[551], antioxidants, antiproliferation[552], chemopreventive[553], gene protective, neuroprotective, pro-oxidant[554]

## Food Sources
- Acai oil, apples, black berries, black grape with skins, cherry, *cocoa, *dark chocolate[555], grapes with skins, *green tea, kola nut, peach, pears, raisins, red wine vinegar

# Epigallocatechin

## Possible Uses
- Alzheimer's[556], anxiety[557], breast cancer[558], cardiovascular disease[559], cervical cancer[560], cholesterol control, chronic fatigue syndrome[561], dementia[562], depression, diabetes (type 2)[563], endometriosis[564], food-borne pathogen, energy, HIV[565], mental health problems[566], neurodegenerative disorders[567], obesity[568], Parkinson's[569], prostate cancer[570], spinal muscular atrophy[571], Sjögren's syndrome[572], weight reduction

## Possible Benefits
- Higher in antioxidants than vitamins C and E.
- Reduces R plasmid transfer of Escherichia coli.[573]

## Properties
- Anti-angiogenic[574], anti-apoptotic, anti-atherosclerotic[575], anti-inflammatory, anticancer, antimicrobial, antioxidant, antiviral

## Warning, Precautions and Side Effects
- Green tea might cause colon damage.[576]

## Food Sources
- Carob flour, cranberry (raw), Fuji apples, hazelnuts, pistachios, tea (*green, Oolong), pecans, St. John's Wort

# Flavonols

## Different Types of Flavonols
  • Gingerol, isorhamnetin, kaempferol, myricetin, quercetin, rutin

## Research
Chocolate and cocoa, high-flavanol foods, are antioxidants and have anti-inflammatory properties as well as aids in cardiovascular protection.[577]


# Gingerol

## Possible Uses
  • Asthma, breast cancer[578], cholesterol control, chronic rheumatic pain, colds, colon cancer[579], colorectal cancer[580], coughs, dementia[581], diarrhea, digestion, gastric cancer[582], gonarthritis (knee), leukemia[583], liver cancer[584], lung cancer[585], morning sickness, motion sickness, nausea, ovarian cancer[586], pancreatic cancer[587], prostate cancer[588], prostatic inflammation[589], rheumatism, rheumatoid arthritis[590], skin cancer[591], stomach upset, ulcers (Helicobacter pylori)[592], vomiting

## Possible Benefits
  • Cooking ginger changes gingerol to zingerone, sweeter.
  • Drying ginger  makes gingerol twice as pungent.
  • Can drop body temperature.
  • Potent nitric oxide (NO) inhibitor.
  • Accentuates airway hyperresponsiveness with asthma[593].

## Properties

- Anti-inflammatory, anticancer, antifungal, antileukemia[594], antioxidant, antiproliferation, antitumor, chemopreventive, pro-apoptotic

## Warning, Precautions, and Side Effects

- Do not use if pregnant, may cause miscarriage.

## Food Sources

- Ginger

## Pain Folk Remedy

- Ginger powder
- Clove powder
- Mix together in water, then rub on pain

## Isorhamnetin

- Metabolite of quercetin.

## Possible Uses

- Arteriosclerosis[595], breast cancer[596], cardiovascular disease[597], cholesterol control, colon cancer[598], diabetes[599], diabetic cataracts[600], esophageal cancer[601], HIV-1[602], heart disease, hypertension, ischaemic stroke[603], leukemia[604], liver cancer, lung cancer[605], non-Hodgkin's lymphoma[606], obesity, osteoporosis, prostate cancer[607], skin cancer[608], skin inflammation, stroke[609]

## Properties

- Anti-inflammatory, antioxidant, antiproliferative, antitumor[610], cytotoxicity[611], hepatoprotective[612]

## Food Sources

- Almonds, beets, broad beans (fava), broccoli, Brussels sprouts, cabbage, carrots, cauliflower, celery, Chinese kale, chives, cucumber, dill, dishcloth gourd, endive, fennel leaves, gingko, honey, kale, kidney beans, kohlrabi, leeks, lettuce, mustard leaf/seed, **onions (spring, white, yellow), parsley, parsnips, peas, peppers, potatoes, radishes, **red onions, sea buckthorn, snap beans, spinach, turnip greens, Vitex negundo L.,watercress, water spinach

## Research

- Hot air-dried onions showed a strong cell proliferated action, but freeze-dried and vacuum-dried only showed moderate on leukemia cells.[613]

## Kaempferol

- Often partnered with Quercetin.

## Possible Uses

- Allergic asthma[614], Alzheimer's[615], arteriosclerosis, cancer[616], breast cancer[617], cardiovascular disease[618], cataracts[619], chronic inflammation disease[620], colon cancer[621], diabetes eye health, diabetes pancreatic damage[622], diabetic cataract[623], eye health [624], gastic cancer [625], HIV-1[626], heart health[627], ischaemic stroke[628], liver cancer[629], liver damage, lung non-small cancer[630], methicillin-resistant Staphylococcus aureus (MRSA)[631], non-Hodgkin's lymphoma[632], oral cancer[633], osteoporosis, ovarian cancer[634], pancreatic cancer[635], Parkinson's[636], prostate cancer[637], stimulates liver detox, stomach cancer[638], stroke

**Possible Benefits**
- Flavonoids are neuroprotective agents for retinal ganglion cells.[639]

**Properties**
- Analgesic, anti-estrogenic, anti-inflammatory, anticancer, anticoagulant, antimicrobial[640], antioxidant, antitumor, cardioprotective, chemopreventive, hypoglycemic, inhibits angiogenesis, low cytotoxicity, neuroprotective[641]

**Food Sources**
- Apricot, beets, belimbi fruit, bird chili, black tea, blackberry, broad beans (fava), broccoli, Brussels sprouts, cabbage, canned capers, carrot, cassia siamea lam stem bark, cauliflower, celery, *Chinese kale, chives, cranberry, cress, cucumber, dill, dishcloth gourd, dock, dried asam gelugur, endive, fava beans, French beans, garlic, *gingko biloba, gooseberry, grape, green chili, green snap beans, guava, kale, kidney beans, kohlrabi, leeks, lettuce, limau purut leaves, local celery, **onion (spring, white, yellow), onion leaves, papaya shoots, parsley, parsnips, peas, peppers, Phaleria microfarad fruit (Crown of God, pau), pomegranate, potato, radishes, red beets, **red onion, rutabagas, scallions, Semambu leaves, snap beans, spinach, strawberries, tea, tomato, tomato products, turnip greens, watercress, water spinach, witch hazel, white radish, yellow snap beans
- Most foods should be raw to maintain integrity.

# Myricetin

## Possible Uses

- Alzheimer's[642], blood sugar control, bone health, breast cancer[643], Burkholderia cepacia multi-drug resistant bacteria[644], cardiovascular disease[645], cholesterol control, colon cancer[646], colorectal cancer[647], diabetes[648], diarrhea, esophageal cancer[649], fever, HIV-1[650], ischaemic stroke[651], leukemia[652], liver cancer[653], lung cancer[654], non-Hodgkin's lymphoma[655], osteoporosis[656], ovarian cancer[657], pancreatic cancer[658], Parkinson's[659], prostate cancer[660], skin cancer, smoker's cessation, Synovial sarcoma rheumatoid arthritis[661], vancomycin-resistant enterococci (VRE)[662]

## Possible Benefits

- Protects DNA from damage.

## Properties

- Anti-inflammatory, anticancer, antioxicant, antitumor, cytotoxic[663], estrogenic

## Food Sources

- Abelmoschus moschatus, bayberry, beets, berries, belimbi fruit, bilberry, black currants, blueberry, bog whortleberry, broad bean, broccoli, Brussels sprouts, cabbage, carrot, cauliflower, celery, *Chinese kale, cranberry, crowberry, cucumber, dishcloth gourd, dock, dried asam gelugur, endive, fava beans, French beans, garlic, green chili, kale, kidney beans, kohlrabi, leeks, lettuce, lemon juice, limau purut leaves, local celery, Myrica cerifera, **onions (spring, white, yellow), parsley, parsnips, peas, peppers, potatoes, radishes, *rutabagas, red grapes or wine, **red onions, snap beans, spinach, sweet potato, tea, tomato, turnip greens, walnuts, watercress, water spinach, white radish

# Quercetin

- Often partnered with Kaempferol.
- Flavonoid aglycone of rutin.

## Possible Uses

- Allergies[664], Alzheimer's[665], angina[666], anxiety[667], atherosclerosis[668], arthritis[669], asthma[670], bone health, bone marrow inflammation[671], breast cancer[672], bursitis, cancer prevention, cancer treatment, cardiovascular disease[673], cataracts[674], cholesterol control, chronic fatigue syndrome[675], chronic obstructive pulmonary disease (COPD)[676], colon cancer[677], Crohn's disease[678], depression, diabetes[679], diabetic cataracts, diabetic neuropathy[680], diabetic retinopathy, digestion, dust allergies, fatigue, fibromyalgia[681], glaucoma, gouty arthritis (gout)[682], HIV-1[683], hay fever, Helicobacter pylori bacteria[684], hives, inflammation[685], inflammatory bowel disease (IBD)[686], ischaemic stroke[687], ischemia/reperfusion induced renal injury[688], leaky gut syndrome[689], leukemia[690] (ALL, APL, CML), liver [691], lung cancer[692], methicillin-resistant Staphylococcus aureus (MRSA),[693], non-Hodgkin's lymphoma[694], mouth sores, neuropathy, osteoporosis[695], ovarian cancer[696], pancreas[697], Parkinson's[698], prostate, prostate cancer[699], prostatitis swelling, reduces pain, Salmonella[700], sinus infection, stomach cancer[701], ulcerated colitis

## Possible Benefits

- Use with bromelein to enhance absorption.
- Strengthens blood vessels.
- Inhibits blood clot formation.
- Aids in blocking HSP expression for eye protection.
- Blocks antigen-stimulated release of histamines, takes several weeks to work.

- Blocks sorbitol, associated with eye, kidney and nerve damage in diabetics.[702]

## Properties

- Anti-artherogenic[703], anti-inflammatory[704], antibacterial, anticancer[705], anti-cytogenotoxic, antihistamine, antimicrobial, antimutagenic, antioxidant, antiplatelet[706], apoptotic, antiproliferative[707], antitumor, anxiolytic[708], cognitive-enhancing effects[709], catatonic, hepatotoxicity, hypolipemic[710]

## Food Sources

- Apricots, beets, belimbi fruit, bilberry, bird chili, black currant, black tea, blue-green algae, blueberry, bog whortleberry, broccoli, Brussel sprouts, buckwheat, cabbage, canned capers, carrot, cauliflower, celery, chamomile (German), cherry, Chinese kale, chokecherry, citrus white material under peel, coriander, cranberry, crowberry, cucumber, dock, dill, dishcloth gourd, dried asam gelugur, endive, fava beans, French beans, garlic, gooseberry,  grapes, green beans, green chili, green tea, gingko biloba, guava, *kale, kidney beans, kohlrabi, leafy green vegetables, leeks, limau purut leaves, local celery, longanberry, lotus leaf extract, lovage, **onion (spring, white, yellow), onion leaves, papaya shoots, parsley, parsnips, peas, peppers, potatoes, prickly pear cactus, raspberry, red apple skin, red cabbage, red grapes, red *onions, red wine, rowanberry, *rutabagas, S buxifolia, sea buckthorn berry, Semambu leaves, snap beans, spinach, St. John's Wort, sea buckthorn berry, spinach, strawberry, sweet potato leaves, sweet rowan, tea, tomato, turnip greens, watercress, water spinach, white radish

## Research

It inhibits Helicobacter pylori growth which is thought to cause peptic ulcers.  It also helps to reduce the effects of Epstein-Barr virus (a common virus; a common cause of mononucleosis), the herpes virus, and the polio virus.[711]

# Rutin

## Possible Uses

* Aging, allergies, Alzheimer's[712], arteriosclerosis[713], arthritis[714], asthma, bleeds easily, blood pressure control[715], breast cancer[716], bruising, CNS dysfunction, cancer, candida[717], cardiovascular disease[718], cataracts, cholesterol control, chronic venous insufficiency[719], circulation, colds, colorectal carcinogenesis[720], congestion, dementia, diabetic retinopathy[721], diabetes[722], dyslipidemia[723], ethanol induced gastric lesions[724], excessive bruising, fatty liver disease[725], flu, gastrointestinal diseases, glaucoma[726], hay fever, headache, heart disease[727], hemorrhagic diseases[728], hemorrhoids, hepatosteatosis[729], high fever, inflammation[730], hypercholesterolemia[731], hyperglycemia[732], hypertension, inflammatory bowel disease (IBD)[733], internal bleeding, iron chelation, Ischemia-reperfusion brain injury and related disorders[734], liver cirrhosis, low serum calcium, memory retrieval[735], metastatic melanoma[736], obesity[737], oral herpes, osteoarthritis, periodontal disease, poor circulation, pre-cancer, prostate cancer[738], radiation[739], radiation sickness[740], rheumatoid arthritis[741], septic arthritis[742], sinusitis, skin care, skin collagen, spider veins, sporadic dementia[743], stress, strokes[744], stomach upset, tardive dyskenisia[745], thrombosis[746], triglyceride level control[747], varicose veins, vascular function[748], venous edema, wrinkles, yeast infections

- Inflammation of the veins in the anus and rectum.

**Possible Benefits**
- Enhance absorption of vitamin C
- Inhibits platelet aggregation
- Potent free radical scavenger.
- Strengthens capillaries and stabilizes capillary walls, making less likely to bleed
- Rutin and hesperidin enhance use of calcium, magnesium, vitamins and minerals
- Bioflavonoid works with vitamin C assists in reducing pain and intraocular pressure
- Protects against damage by antibiotics, aspirin, and cortisone
- In hemorrhagic diseases, it decreases capillary fragility.[749]
- Decreases vessel permeability.[750]
- Prevents blood clot formation.[751]
- Most effective in chronic arthritis.
- Stimulates bone marrow production.
- Can help prevent blood clots.

**Properties**
- Anti-arthritis[752], anti-inflammatory[753], anticancer, anticandida[754], anticarcinogenic, anticonvulsant[755], antiedema[756], antifungal[757], antioxidant, antiplatelet[758], antitumor, excellent electrochemical activity[759], metal chelator, neuroprotective[760], radioprotective[761]

**Warning, Precautions and Side Effects**
- Dizziness, fatigue, headache, heart racing, muscle stiffness, stomach upset
- Allergic reactions are breathing problems, chest pain, skin rashes, swelling

**Food Sources**

- Apples and peel, *apricot, asparagus, berries, blackberry, blueberry, broccoli, *buckwheat (kasha), *cherries, *citrus fruit, citrus white part of peel, cranberry, garlic, grapefruit, grapes, green peppers, green tea (warning in Other Info), lemons, lime, onions, mulberry fruit (functional food)[762], nettle, noni, orange, peaches, plums, prunes, red apple skin, red raspberry, rhubarb, rue (herb-of-grace), sophora japonica, tea (black, green, yerba mate), tomato, Vietnamese cauliflower
- The leaves and petioles of Rheum species and asparagus.
- Buckwheat is the only field crop to contain rutin, not found in other grains such as beans, rice, wheat.
- The tablet form supplement is best because it's rare to get the needed amount in natural foods.

**Research**

Robert Flaumenhalf, associate professor at Harvard Medical School, stated that rutin is an unbeatable compound, that this one single agent can inhibit platelet accumulation in the arteries and fibrin generation in the veins and would make a inexpensive, safe, new drug.[763]

When dealing with rheumatoid arthritis, rutin became very active in the chronic stage.[764]

# Flavones

**Three types of flavones.**
- Apigenin, luteolin, and tangeritin.


# Apigenin

- Citrus bioflavonoid

**Possible Uses**
- Alzheimer's[765], anxiety neurosis[766], atherosclerosis, breast cancer[767], candida albicans, cardiovascular disease[768], cerebral artery occusion-induced focal ischemia[769], colon cancer[770], digestive tract cancer[771], hematological malignancies[772], hypermononoaminergic neuropsychological disorders[773], learning and memory[774], leukemia[775], lowers body fat, lung cancer[776], lymphoma[777], neurodegenerative diseases[778], neurological disease[779], non-Hodgkin's lymphoma[780], obesity[781], oral cancer[782], Parkinson's[783], Promyelocytic leukemia HL-60[784], prostate cancer[785], renal damage from cyclosporin[786], respiratory syncytial virus[787], seizures[788], skin cancer[789]

**Possible Benefits**
- Might have neurogenesis in which neurons are created and might be useful for neurological diseases.[790]
- Potent inhibitor of CYP2C9, a mediator for drug-to-drug interactions.[791]

## Properties

- Anti-adipogenic, anti-inflammatory, antibacterial, anticancer[792], antileukemic, antioxidant, antiplatelet[793], antiproliferative, antiviral[794], anxiolytic[795], apoptotic[796], chemopreventive, cytopathic[797], hepatoprotective[798], neuroprotective[799]

- Rosa damascena, a flavor and fragrance, is considered to be anti-HIV, antibacterial, anticonvulsant, antispasmodic, antioxidant, antitussive, anxielytic, choleretic, hepatoprotective, hypnotic, laxative, relaxant and confirmed to be safe.[800]

## Food Sources

- Bell pepper, broad bean (fava), broccoli, Brussel sprouts, cabbage, cauliflower, *celery, celery seed, citrus, citrus flower, Chinese cabbage, Chinese kale, dishcloth gourd, daun turi, French peas, fruits, garlic, grapefruit, guava, kadok, kohlrabi, lettuce, licorice, local celery, marjoram, onion leaves, oregano, *parsley, peppermint, peppers, Perilla frutescens (L) Britt[801], petroselinum crispum extract[802], prosthechea michuacana orchid, red wine, rosa damascena[803], rosemary, rutabagas, snake gourd, spinach, tarragon, thyme, tomato sauce, turnera aphrodisiaca, water spinach, wolfberry

# Luteolin

- Yellow compound in leaves.

## Possible Uses

- ADD/ADHD[804], allergies, Alzheimer's[805], Aspergers[806], atherosclerosis[807], autism[808], B. subtilis[809], Bacillus cereus[810], blood sugar control, bone loss[811], cancer[812], breast cancer[813], cancer[814], candida albicans[815], chemotherapy, cognition[816], colon cancer[817], Cryptococcus neoformans[818], eczema, Escherichia coli[819], gamma ($\gamma$)-irradiation pretreatment[820], gastric hypersecretion[821], gastritis[822], gram positive/negative organisms, HIV-1[823], heart disease, hypermononoaminergic neuropsychological disorders[824], immune disorders, Klebsiella pneumoniae[825], learning[826], memory[827], mercury-induced toxicity pretreatment[828], multiple sclerosis[829], nausea, neurodegenerative diseases[830], non-Hodgkin's lymphoma[831], osteoporosis[832], ovarian cancer[833], Parkinson's[834], prostate cancer[835], Pseudomonas aeruginosa[836], reflux esophagitis[837], rheumatoid arthritis[838], skin cancer[839], Staphylococcus aureus[840], UV-B radiation[841], ulcers[842]

## Possible Benefits

- Crosses the blood brain barrier.
- Therapeutic compound that poisons topoisomerases in cancer.[843]

## Properties

- Analgesic, anti-allergy, anti-inflammatory, antibacterial[844], anticancer, antifungal[845], antihistamine, antimicrobial[846], antioxidant, antichloristic, antiproliferation, antitumor[847], apoptotoxic, chemopreventive, neuroprotective, spasmolytic

**Warning, Precautions and Side Effects**
- Monitor intake of luteolin with allergies, asthma and chronic obstructive pulmonary disease (COPD), nausea and vomiting.[848]

**Food Sources**
- Artichoke leaves extract, Bacopa monnieri species[849], belimbi fruit, bird chili, black tea, carrot, *celery, chamomile, Chinese kale, citrus, dandelion, beets, Brussels sprouts, cabbage, cauliflower, dishcloth gourd, kidney beans, naval oranges, *olive leaf extract, *olive oil, oregano, papaya shoots, **parsley, peppermint, peppers, Perilla frutescens (L) Britt[850], *pomegranate, propolis, Semambu leaves, spinach, thyme, water spinach, white radish, wild lettuce, yarrow

**Research**
The environmental neurotoxin HgCL2 (mercury choloride) is used in vaccines as a preservative. Use of luteolin 10 minutes before the vaccine blocked HgCL2's effects. Mercury toxicity can also be blocked with methyl thiosalicylate and luteolin.[851]

## Tangeritin

- Often partnered with nobiletin, which is also from tangerine peels.
- Citrus flavonoid can cross the blood brain barrier.

### Possible Uses
- Alzheimer's[852], atherosclerosis[853], avian influenza H5N1[854], breast cancer[855], candida albicans, cardiovascular disease[856], cholesterol control, colon cancer[857], congestion, dementia[858], dispels mucus, dysentery, dyspepsia, fever, HIV[859], hair loss, heart palpitations, hemorrhoids[860], influenza[861], intestinal tumor[862], Kirsten murine sarcoma virus deterant[863], leukemia[864], lung cancer[865], metastatic melanoma[866], neurodegenerative diseases[867], ovarian cancer[868], Parkinson's[869], prostate cancer (minor support), restenosis[870], skin repair

### Properties
- Antibacterial, anticancer, antifungal, antileukemic[871], antimicrobial, antioxidant, antiproliferation, antitumor, chemopreventive[872], neuroprotective

### Warning, Precautions, and Side Effects
- Can interfere with tamoxifen and other medications. Check with your physician.

### Food Sources
- Clementine peels, garlic, Mandarin orange peels, some citrus peels, tangerine peels

# Flavanones      Isoflavones

- Estrogen-like effects found in bean/legume family.

## Different Types of Flavanones/Isoflavones
- Eriodictyol, hesperidin, naringenin, silybin.

# Eriodictyol

- Often paired with luteolin but more often used with other flavonoids.
- Citrus falconoid can cross the blood brain barrier.

## Possible Uses
- Breast cancer[873], cancer[874], cholesterol control[875], melanoma[876], Ménière's disease[877], prostate, tinnitus (ear ringing), vasodilatory[878], virtigo and hearing improvement[879]

## Possible Benefits
- Inhibits neoplastic cell transformation.
- Improves cellular defenses to inhibit oxidative injury.

## Properties
- Anti-apoptotic, anti-inflammatory, antimicrobial, antioxidant, antiplatelet, antiproliferative, antiproteasomal, antiprotozoan[880], antitumor, cytoprotective[881],

## Food Sources

- Bergamot (citrus bergamia risso), citrus fruits, eureka lemon, koji (citrus leiocarpa), grapefruit, lumie fruit(highest), oranges, sambokan (citrus sulcata), sudachi (citrus sudachi) Yerba Santa

## Research

Out of 27 citrus falconoid, seven were found to have antiproliferative activities against human tumor cells. They are eriodictyol, luteolin (highest), natsudaidain, quercetin, tangeretin and nobiletin (lowest).[882]

# Hesperidin

- Citrus falconoid can cross the blood brain barrier.

## Possible Uses

- Abnormal capillary leakiness[883], aches/pain[884], aging skin care[885], allergies, androgen-dependant prostate cancer[886], Alzheimer's[887], arthritis[888], autoimmune diseases, avian flu, blood pressure control, bone loss[889], bone quality, breast cancer[890], cancer, candida yeast infection[891], cardiovascular disease[892], cholesterol control, chronic pain[893], collagen-induced arthritis[894], colon cancer[895], diabetes (type 2)[896], edema in legs (fluid retention), hay fever, hypertension[897], immune system stimulant, influenza (H5N1)[898], influenza A (H1N1)[899], leg cramps[900], lung cancer[901], menopause, night leg cramps[902], multiple sclerosis[903], osteoporosis[904], Parkinson's[905], rheumatoid arthritis[906], sepsis syndrome[907], memory, weakness[908], stroke[909], wrinkles[910]

## Possible Benefits of Hesperidin

- Contributes to the integrity of the blood vessels.

- Aids in increasing bone mineral density, bone strength.[911]
- Large doses of the glucoside hesperidin decreased bone density loss in mice.
- Hesperidin and rutin may aid in reducing capillary permeability.
- Hesperidin and rutin may also have anti-inflammatory effects.
- Works with vitamin C to maintain collagen.

## Properties

- Analgesic, anti-allergen, anti-infection, anti-inflammatory, anticancer, antifungal, antihistamine, antinociceptive, antioxidant, antispasmodic, antitumor[912], antiviral, depurative, hypoglycemic, hypolipidemic, neuroprotective, nutrigenomic, refrigerant, sedative, stimulant, UVR protectant[913]

## Warnings, Precautions, and Side Effects

- Do not use if hypersensitive to it or to any hesperidin-containing products.
- Pregnant women and nursing mothers should avoid high doses, unless approved by their doctor.
- May cause nausea and other gastrointestinal problems.

## Possible Supplemental Usage

- Rutin and hesperidin improve the utilization of calcium, magnesium, along with all vitamins and minerals.

## Food Sources

- Citrus fruits, pulp & rind, grapefruit seed extract, orange peel

# Naringenin

- Citrus falconoid can cross the blood brain barrier.

**Possible Uses**
- Alzheimer's[914], amnesia[915], anxiety[916], atherosclerosis[917], breast cancer[918], cancer, cholesterol control[919], colon cancer[920], coronary artery disease[921], depression[922], diabetes[923], ethanol-induced hepatotoxicity[924], heart disease[925], hepatitis C virus[926], Huntington's[927], hyperinsulinemia[928], lung metastasis with fibrosis[929], non-small cell lung cancer[930], obesity[931], Parkinson's[932], prostate cancer[933]

**Possible Benefits**
- Stimulates DNA repair.[934]

**Properties**
- Anti-atherogenic[935], anti-inflammatory, anticancer, antidepressant[936], antioxidant, antitumor[937], antineoplasic against multidrug-resistant cancer cells[938], anxiolytic[939], neuroprotective[940], proliferative[941]

**Food Sources**
- Citrus fruits, grapefruit, lemons, limes, orange, tangerines

# Silybin / Silymarin

- Silybin is pure chemical and silymarin is the flavononoid complex from milk thistle seeds.
- Crosses blood brain barrier.

## Possible Uses

- AIDS dementia[942], acute myeloid leukemia (AML)[943], alcoholic/non steatohepatitis, allergic asthma[944], Alzheimer's[945], amanita death cap mushroom poisoning[946], amyloid $\beta$ peptide-induced memory impairment[947], bladder cancer[948], breast cancer[949], CNS diseases[950], cardio-pulmonary problems[951], chronic hepatitis C[952], chronic liver disease[953], colon cancer[954], colorectal cancer, diabetes (type 2)[955], fibrosarcoma[956], gastrointestinal problems[957], kidney chemical-induced injury[958], liver cancer[959], liver cirrhosis[960], lung tumor[961], memory, nephropathy[962], nonalcoholic fatty liver disease[963], ovarian cancer[964], pancreas recovery[965], Parkinson's[966], prostate cancer[967], skin cancer[968], skin health, UV skin protection[969]

## Possible Benefits
- Doesn't have undesirable side effects.
- Doesn't seem to interact with other drugs.

## Properties
- Anti-inflammatory, antibacterial, anticancer[970], antifibrotic, antineoplastic, antioxidant, antiproliferation, antitumor, antiviral (CNS)[971], chemopreventive, chemotherapeutic[972], cytoprotective[973], drug transporter[974], estrogenic[975], hepatoprotective[976], neuro-immunomodulation[977] neuroprotective, neuroprotective, neurotropic

**Food Sources**

- Artichokes, milk thistle seeds has both silybin and silymarin.

**Research**

Research studies show that silybin seems to be more bioavailability than silymarin.[978]

Over 12,000 papers have been written in the last 10 years which don't appear to substantiate clearly to recommend its usage.[979]

# Lignans    Phytoestrogens

- Estrogen-like plant chemical compound.

## Types of Lignans (phytoestrogens)
- Hydroxymatairesinol, lariciresinol, matairesinol, pinoresino, secoisolariciresinol, sesamin, solitarian, syringaresinol

The last two types of lignans will not be discussed.

## High Dietary Lignan Foods

### Possible Uses
- Alzheimer's[980], breast cancer[981], cardiovascular disease[982], colon cancer[983], colorectal cancer[984], coronary heart disease[985], diabetes (type 2)[986], endometrium[987], heart disease[988], lung ischemia-reperfusion injury[989], menopausal symptoms[990], neurological problems, osteoporosis[991], ovarian cancer[992],  ovarian hormone deficiency[993], prostate cancer[994], stroke[995]

### Properties
- Acts like an antioxidant, apoptotic, antiumor[996], cytostatic, diuretic, phototropic ()creosote

### Highest Lignan Food Sources
- Flaxseed[997] and sesame seed

### Other Lignan Food Sources
- Creosote bush Larrea tridentata (Zygophyllaceae)

**Research**

Lariciresinol, matairesinol, ingression and secoisolariciresinol can reduce the risk of cardiovascular disease and specific cancers because of enterolignans (enterodiol and enterolactone) precursers, which after eating lignans, form intestinal microflora. The richest is flaxseed, then sesame seed.[998]

## Hydroxymatairesinol

- Produced by intestinal bacteria from fiber-rich diets.

**Possible Uses**

- AIDS/HIV[999], Alzheimer's[1000], breast cancer[1001], cardiovascular disease[1002], colorectal cancer[1003], coronary heart disease[1004], ENNG-uterine carcinogenesis[1005], estrogen-dependant diseases, Parkinson's[1006], prostate cancer[1007]

**Properties**

- Antitumor[1008], chemopreventive

**Food Sources**

- Barley bran, flaxseed, *Norway spruce (Picea abies) heartwood, oat bran, rye bran, *sesame seed, wheat bran,

**Research**

In the 2006, the US Patent for "METHOD OF INHIBITING OVERACTIVITY OF PHAGOCYTES OR LYMPHOCTES IN AN INDIVIDUAL" states that it might be helpful in treating inflammatory bowel conditions, AIDS/HIV, Alzheimer's, autoimmune conditions, Parkinson's, and psoriasis. Hydroxymatairesinol and Matairesinol are in the patent.[1009]

# Lariciresinol

## Possible Uses
- Alzheimer's[1010], breast cancer[1011], candida albicans[1012], cardiovascular disease[1013], colorectal cancer[1014], diabetes (type 2)[1015], estrogen deficiency[1016], HIV, mammary cancer[1017], ovarian cancer[1018], Parkinson's[1019], prostate cancer[1020], ulcers[1021]

## Properties
- anticancer, antifungal, antioxidant, antitumor[1022], antiulcer[1023]

## Food Sources
- Araucaria araucana (Mol) K Koch, barley bran, brassica vegetables, English/Eruopean yew (Taxus baccata L)[1024], flaxseed, Korean barberry (Berberes koreana)[1025], oat bran, rye bran, sambucus williamsii, *sesame seeds, wheat bran

# Matairesinol

## Possible Uses
- AIDS/HIV[1026], Alzheimer's[1027], asthma[1028], bone loss[1029], breast cancer[1030], cancer[1031], cardiovascular disease (CVD)[1032], cardiovascular health[1033], chronic obstructive pulmonary disease[1034], coronary heart disease (CHD)[1035], diabetes (type 2)[1036], lung disease[1037], osteoporosis[1038], ovarian cancer[1039], Parkinson's[1040], prostate cancer[1041], stroke[1042], vascular inflammation[1043]

## Properties
- Anti-inflammatory, anticancer, antimicrobial, antioxidant, immunomodulator

**Food Sources**
- Barley bran, blackcurrants, broccoli, flax seeds, oat bran, rye bran, sea buckthorn, *sesame seeds, strawberries, wheat bran

## Pinoresinol

**Possible Uses**
- Alzheimer's[1044], atherosclerosis[1045], cardiovascular disease[1046], colon cancer[1047], coronary heart disease, diabetes (type 2)[1048], estrogen deficiency[1049], HIV[1050], hypertension[1051], multiple sclerosis[1052], neurodegenerative disease[1053], prostate cancer[1054], stroke[1055]

**Properties**
- Anti-inflammatory, antifungal, antimalarial, antioxidant, antiproliferative, hepatoprotective

**Food Sources**
- Barley bran, brassica vegetables, Eucommia extract (olive bark)[1056], flaxseed, Forsythia koreana[1057], Forsythiae Fructus, oat bran, olive oil, rye bran, **sesame seeds, wheat bran

# Secoisolariciresinol

## Possible Uses
- Alzheimer's[1058], amyotrophic lateral sclerosis[1059], atherosclerosis[1060], benign prostatic hyperplasia[1061], bone density, breast cancer[1062], cataract[1063], cervical cancer[1064], colon cancer[1065], colorectal cancer[1066], coronary heart disease[1067], diabetes (type 1)[1068], (type 2)[1069], HIV[1070], hormone-related cancer[1071], hypercholesterolemia[1072], ischemic heart disease[1073], liver cancer[1074], liver disease[1075], memory loss[1076], multiple sclerosis[1077], obesity, ovarian cancer[1078], Parkinson's, prostate cancer[1079], rheumatic diseases[1080]

## Properties
- anticancer, antitumor[1081], antioxidant, antitumor[1082], apoptotic[1083], cytostatic[1084]

## Food Sources
- Barley bran, blueberry, cranberry, **flax seed, garlic, oat bran, onions, pumpkin seed, rye bran, sea buckthorn, sesame seed, stereospermum personatum[1085], strawberry, sunflower seed, wheat bran

# Sesamin

## Possible Uses

- Alzheimer's[1086], arterial wall fibrinoid degeneration[1087], breast cancer[1088], cerebral thrombogenesis[1089], chronic disease[1090], conjunctivitis, colon cancer[1091], connective tissue preservation[1092], coronary heart disease, HIV, hyperlipidemia[1093], hypertension, influenza A (H1N1)[1094], influenza virus A neuraminidase[1095], leukemia tumor cells[1096], liver damage[1097], lowers liver and serum cholesterol[1098], lung cancer[1099], multiple myeloma[1100], neurodegenerative diseases[1101], pancreas cancer [1102], Parkinson's[1103], prostate cancer[1104], renal damage[1105], salt-loaded hypertension[1106], stroke[1107]

## Possible

- Decreased liver fatty acid synthesis.[1108]
- Increased DHA concentrations in Alzheimer's disease.[1109]

## Properties

- Anti-inflammatory[1110], anticytokine storm[1111], antidegenerative, antihypertensive[1112], antimicrobial, antimitotic, antioxidant, antitumor[1113], antiviral[1114], chemoprotective[1115], neuroprotective[1116]

## Food Sources

- Sesame seed

# Terpenes   (isoprenoids)

## Carotenoids    (tetraterpenoids)

There are 5 types of carotenoids
• α-Carotene, β-Carotene, lycopene, phytoene, and phytofluene

• Fat soluble organic plant pigment.
• Can fight chronic diseases.
• Can be found in some algae, bacteria, and fungus.
• Cannot be made by animals.
• Acts as an antioxidant.

### Alpha Carotene       α-Carotene

• Fat soluble.
• Precursor to Retinol.

**Possible Uses**
   • Age-related macular degeneration[1117], Alzheimer's disease[1118], asthma[1119], atherosclerosis[1120], breast cancer[1121], cancer, cataracts, cervical cancer, cervical dysphasia, chronic obstructive pulmonary disease (COPD)[1122], colon cancer[1123], HIV[1124], heart disease[1125], male infertility[1126], osteoarthritis, photosensitivity, prostate cancer[1127]

**Possible Benefits**
   • Provitamin A compound, converted into retinol.
   • Stimulates cell to cell communication.

**Properties**
   • Anti-aging, antioxidant, antiproliferative

---

## Warning, Precautions, and Side Effects
- People on a low-fat diet may cause digestive tract absorption problems.
- Smokers and drinkers may have low levels of alpha-carotene.
- Smokers and drinkers should consult physician before supplementing with a carotenoid.

## Food Sources
- Yellow-orange and dark green vegetables.
- Apples, avocado, broccoli, cantaloupe, carrots, cilantro, collards, green beans, green peas, kale, leaf lettuce, maize, orange, pumpkin, romaine lettuce, spinach, sweet potatoes, Swiss chard, tangerine, thyme (fresh), tomatoes, turnip greens, winter squash

## Beta Carotene     β-Carotene

## What is beta-carotene?
- A dietary chemical which changes into and supplies vitamin A.
- Fat soluble.
- Foods produce colors in the orange and yellow range.
- Rich foods may be other colors also, such as pink, red, purple, white and dark leafy green and yellow vegetables.
- Helps reproductive system perform correctly.
- Quick intervention of a person with cancer with heavy dosages of beta-carotene, the greater the likelihood tumor development won't occur.

## Possible Uses

- AIDS[1128], acne, age-related macular degeneration[1129], Alzheimer's[1130], anemia, anti-aging, antioxidant, asthma, benign prostatic hyperplasia[1131], blindness, bone growth, bone strength, breast cancer[1132], bronchitis, cancer, cardiovascular disease[1133], cataracts, cervical cancer[1134], cervical dysphasia[1135], colorectal cancer[1136], Cystic Fibrosis[1137], dermatitis, diarrhea, diabetes (type 2)[1138], digestion, dry rough skin(goose flesh), embryonic (fetus) development, eye health, female infertility, female organs, fatigue, gastric cancer[1139], HIV[1140], healthy fetus, immune system, infectious diseases, keratomalacia[1141], lactation, liver problems, macular degeneration[1142], male infertility, measles, night blindness[1143], normal sperm, nutritional blindness[1144], obesity[1145], obstructive pulmonary disease (COPD)[1146], oral leukkoplakia (tobacco/alcohol use oral white lesions), pancreatic cancer[1147], photosensitivity (EPP)[1148], pneumonia, radiation-induced disease[1149], pre-term infant retinopathy[1150], prostate cancer[1151], reproduction, rosacea (+ probiotics)[1152], scleroderma (hardened skin), skin cancer (debated)[1153], skin problems, tumors, UV skin tumors[1154], urinary tract problems, vaginal candida[1155], vision loss[1156], weak teeth, xerophthalmia (cornea drying)[1157]

## Possible Benefits

- High dietary fiber intake reduces body fat.[1158]
- Provitamin A compound, converted into retinol.
- Increases the immune system.
- Free radical scavenger.
- Aids with mucous membrane, skeleton, skin, soft tissue and teeth health.
- Increases cell-to-cell communication.[1159]
- Retinoid precursor.

• Vitamin E and beta-carotene, antioxidants, increase infant defenses against oxygen toxicity through breast-feeding.[1160]

• Aids with healthy epithelial tissue (eyes, GI tract, respiratory, skin, and urinary tract).

## Possible Deficiency

• Requires fat for good absorption throughout the digestive tract, therefore it can be impaired by an extremely low fat diet.

• Crohn's disease, pancreatic enzyme deficiency, celiac sprue, Cystic Fibrosis, or the surgical removal of the gall bladder, stomach, or liver disease, a deficiency of beta carotene may cause a decrease in the body's ability to absorb dietary fat.

• Cigarette smoke kills arytenoids, carotenoid supplements should be used with care because of vitamin A toxicity, see your medical provider.

## Properties

• Antibacterial, anticancer, antioxidant, antitumor, antiviral, chemopreventive[1161]

## Warnings, Precautions, and Side Effects

• Smokers should stay away from beta-carotene supplementation.[1162]

• Pregnant women should use beta-carotene instead of large dosages of vitamin A, which may increase risk of birth defects.

• Pregnant women who are night blind have a likeliness of dying in childbirth from infection to be 5 times greater than those who don't have night blindness.[1163]

• High intake of carotenoid-containing foods are not connected to any toxic side effects.

• Cod liver oil may create toxicity if one doesn't stick to the correct dosage on the label.

• Excessive consumption of beta-carotene can cause a yellowish discoloration of the skin, carotenodermia, reversible and harmless.

• Vitamin A in doses 25,000 units (five times the RDA) of more can lead to blurred vision, hair loss, headaches, and liver damage.[1164]

• A high dosage of 50,000 IU beta-carotene can be used for 1-2 days to treat viral infections.

• European women have reported carotene-containing tanning pills cause infertility.

• Antibiotics, some cholesterol-lowering drugs, and laxative interfere with vitamin A absorption.

• Too much may cause an orange tint to skin which is not harmful.

• Bruising, joint pain, loose stools.

• Can interact with cholestyramin, colestipol, orlistat, and statins medications.

• May cause adverse effects with smokers, may even promote lung cancer[1165] and breast cancer[1166].

• Two research studies show heavy smokers and people who drink alcohol often, might improve their possibility of not developing heart disease and/or lung cancer if they take beta-carotene supplements in a quantity larger than 20-30 milligrams daily.[1167]

• I found studies that recommended that smokers take more beta-carotene and other studies that said if you use it, your risk of death is higher. I think that if you are a smoker, see your physician first, especially before taking vitamin A or beta-carotene supplements.  It's better to err on the side of safety.

**Cooking, Storage and Processing of Beta-carotene**
 • Lightly steamed carrots and spinach improves your body's absorbability of carotenoids, although high heat and/or extended cooking of vegetables decreases the availability of arytenoids.
 • Fresh carrots have 100% all-trans beta-carotene, but canned carrots have only about 70% all-trans beta-carotene.

**Food Sources**
 • Red, yellow-orange and dark green vegetables.
 • Alfalfa, apples, apricots, asparagus, avocado, broccoli, butternut squash, cantaloupe, *carrots, cilantro, collard greens, dandelion greens, dark leafy green vegetables, fresh thyme, green beans, green peppers, kale, lettuce, mangoes, mustard greens, nectarine, nettle, okra, papaya, peach, peas, peppers, *pumpkin, red leaf lettuce, romaine lettuce, spinach, squash, sweet gourd leaves, *sweet potatoes & leaves, tangerine, tomatoes, turnip greens, Vietnamese cauliflower, watercress, watermelon, winter squash, yams
 • Commercially made from algae, fungi, or palm oil.

* **The best of the rest**
| | |
|---|---|
| 1 medium baked sweet potato | 28,805 IU |
| 1/2 c. canned pumpkin | 27,018 IU |
| 1 medium raw carrots | 12,767 IU |

**Research**

A Philadelphia cancer center recommend antioxidants to wage war against malignant mesothelioma. They recommend beta carotene to fight at the cellular level against oxidative stress. Apples, some beans, blueberries, cherries, cranberries, plums, and strawberries are high in antioxidants. There are some drugs based on antioxidants which are used to treat breast cancer, diabetes, lung disease and malaria. But what is really important, the Philadelphia Thomas Jefferson Hospital's Kimmel Cancer Center discovered that these antioxidant drugs are effective against cancers, like mesothelioma.[1168]

Vitamin C, E, beta-carotene and zinc in high dietary intake are recommended for a substantially reduced risk of elderly people getting age-related macular degeneration.[1169]

## Lycopene

- Bright red pigment.

**Possible Uses**

- Age-related macular degeneration, breast cancer[1170], cataracts, cervical cancer[1171], cholesterol control, chronic disease, colon cancer[1172], esophagus cancer[1173], exercise-induced asthma, fibrocystic breast cells[1174], gastric cancer, HIV[1175], heart disease, lung cancer[1176], male fertility[1177], pancreas cancer[1178], pre-term infant retinopathy[1179], oral cavity cancer[1180], ovarian cancer[1181], prostate cancer[1182], rectal cancer[1183], skin cancer, stomach cancer[1184]

## Properties

- Anti-inflammatory, anticancer, antioxidant, antitumor, chemopreventive

## Warning, Precautions and Side Effects

- Lycopene is destroyed in the skin with sun damage, faster than beta carotene.[1185]

## Food Sources

- Apricot, asparagus, basil (dried), canned tomato products, chili powder, cooked tomato products, grapefruit (pink, red), guava, liver, parsley (dried), persimmons, red cabbage, red fruit and vegetables, *tomatoes, watermelon

## Phytoene

- Precursor to Lycopene.[1186]

## Possible Uses

- Age-related mascular degeneration[1187], breast cancer[1188], neurodegenerative diseases, prostate cancer[1189], sunburn[1190]

## Possible Benefits

- Accumulates in our skin and protects it.

## Properties

- Anti-inflammatory, anticancer, anticarcinogenesis[1191], antioxidants, antitumor (UV-B)[1192], chemopreventive, immunomodulator, photoprotective[1193]

**Food Sources**
- Apricots, cantaloupe, Cara Cara orange, mango, orange, papaya, peaches, pink grapefruit, prunes, pumpkin, sweet potato, *tomato, watermelon
- Phytoene accumulates in Cara Cara skin and pulp.

## Phytofluene

- Precursor to Lycopene.[1194]

**Possible Uses**
- Breast cancer[1195], erythematic (UV light)[1196], prostate cancer[1197], UV-B-induced tumors[1198]

**Possible Benefits**
- Accumulates in our skin and protects it.
- Inhibits cancer cell proliferation.

**Properties**
- Anti-inflammatory, anticancer, antioxidant, immunomodulator, photoprotective[1199]

**Food Sources**
- Apricots, cantaloupe, mango, orange, papaya, peaches, pink grapefruit, prunes, pumpkin, star fruit, sweet potato, *tomato, watermelon

# Xanthophylls

There are 4 types of Xanthophylls.
• Astaxanthin, canthaxanthin, cryptoxanthin, lutein and zeaxanthin.


• Marine carotenoids.
• Yellow pigment in leaves, usually masked by chlorophyll.
• Contains oxygen.
• Don't require light for synthesis.
• Captures sunlight wavelengths not captured  by chlorophylls, increasing the visible sunlight spectrum.
• Protects plants from damage with very high radiation.
• Found in all etiolated leaves and young leaves.


## Astaxanthin
## King of Carotenoids

• Fat soluble.
• Crosses the blood brain barrier.
• Crosses blood retinal barrier.
• Red, red/orange pigment.

**Possible Uses**
> • Age-related dementia[1200], age-related macular degeneration[1201], Alzheimer's[1202], Amyotrophic lateral sclerosis (ALS-Lou Gehrig's disease)[1203], anxiety[1204], asthma[1205], atherosclerosis[1206], autoimmune diseases[1207], autoimmune marine lupus[1208], back pain[1209], benign prostate hyperplasia[1210], blood pressure control[1211], breast cancer[1212], cancer[1213], canker sores, cardiovascular disease[1214], carpal tunnel[1215], cataracts[1216],

cholesterol control[1217], chronic inflammatory disease[1218], cognitive function[1219], colon cancer[1220], coloring agent, coronary heart disease[1221], Crohn's[1222], diabetes[1223], diabetic neuropathy[1224], dyspepsia[1225], endurance, fibromyalgia[1226], ganglion cell damage[1227], gastrointestinal problems[1228], glaucoma, HIV[1229], $HgCl_2$-induced acute renal failure[1230], healthy estradiol level[1231], healthy testosterone levels[1232], hepatitis[1233], Huntington's[1234], hyperlipidemia, hypertension, immune system health[1235], insulin-dependant diabetes mellitus[1236], iron chelator, ischemia-reperfusion[1237], joint pain[1238], learning and memory[1239], leukemia[1240], liver[1241], liver disease[1242], male infertility[1243], mammary tumors[1244], menstrual cramps[1245], mercury renal failure[1246], mitochondrial diseases[1247], multiple sclerosis[1248], muscle recovery[1249], neural stem cell proliferation[1250], neurodegenerative disorders[1251], non-alcoholic fatty liver disease[1252], obesity[1253], ocular health[1254], osteoarthritis[1255], PMS[1256], panic disorder[1257], Parkinson's[1258], peptic ulcers[1259], post-surgery inflammation[1260], prostate[1261], psoriasis vulgaris[1262], reflux symptoms[1263], rheumatoid arthritis[1264], senility[1265], skin health[1266], sakin disease[1267], sore muscles[1268], stamina, stroke[1269], thrombosis[1270], transplant rejection[1271], trauma injuries[1272], tuberculosis[1273], UV eye damage[1274], UV skin damage[1275], ulcerative colitis[1276], ulcers[1277], vascular dementia[1278]

## Possible Benefits
- Attaches to cell, protects inside and outside.
- Fights several free radicals by creating an electron cloud which protects the molecule.
- Because it's fat soluble, it's best to take with fish oil.
- Can be 100 times higher in the liver than vitamin E level.[1279]

## Properties

- Anti-aging, anti-anxiety, anti-inflammatory[1280], anticancer, antihypertensive[1281], antimicrobial, antioxidant[1282], antithrombotic, antitumor[1283], antiviral, anxiolytic, chemopreventive, immunostimulant, neuroprotective[1284], photoprotective[1285]

## Food Sources

- Botryococcus braunii, carrots, chlorella zofingiensis, crab crawfish, crustaceans, egg yolks, fish eggs, fungi, krill, lobster, marine algae, microalgae *Haematococcus pluvialis (extract)[1286], propolis, rainbow trout, red peppers, red sea bream, salmon, shellfish, shrimp, Xanthophyllomyces dendrorhous yeast, *wild sockeye salmon
- Red pigmented fruits and vegetables.
- Heating certain foods make the red color visible, like cooking shrimp or lobster.
- There are commercial synthetic sources.

# Canthaxanthin

- Can't be converted into vitamin A.
- Often used with Astaxanthin.

## Possible Uses

- Abdominal obesity[1287], age-related macular degeneration, Alzheimer's, cancer[1288], cardiovascular disease[1289], cholesterol control[1290], coloring agent, erythropoietin protoporphyria (sun sensibivity), food additive, mammary tumors[1291], neurodegenerative disorders[1292], oral carcinogenesis, Parkinson's[1293], prostate cancer[1294], stroke, UV damage[1295]

## Properties

- Anti-inflammatory, anticancer, antioxidant, antiradical, ant photosensitivity, antitumor[1296], chemopreventive, hypocholesterolmic, immunoenhancement of vitamin A, neuroprotective, photoprotective

## Warning, Precautions, and Side Effects

- Do not ingest canthaxanthin in a tanning salon, may cause death by way of aplastic anemia.[1297]
- May cause deposition of retina pigment.

## Food Sources

- Apple peels, carp, crab, crustaceans, eggs, fish, golden mullet, green algae (haematococcus pluvialis), krill, lobster, mushrooms, paprika, phaffia rhodozyma yeast, salmon, shrimp, tanning pills

# Cryptoxanthin
# Beta-Cryptoxanthin

## Possible Uses

- Age-related macular degeneration, Alzheimer's[1298], breast cancer[1299], cancer[1300], cardiovascular disease[1301], colon cancer[1302], coronary artery disease[1303], dementia[1304], diabetes (type 2)[1305], HIV[1306], inflammatory disorders[1307], liver health, lung cancer[1308], lung tumors[1309], myeloid leukemia[1310], non-Hodgkin lymphoma (NHL)[1311], renal cell cancer[1312], rheumatoid arthritis[1313]

## Properties

- Anticancer, antioxidant, chemopreventive

**Food Sources**
- Apple peel, avocado, bovine blood serum, butter, egg yolk, flower and rose petals (Physalis), food coloring, grapefruit, kiwi, mandarin orange juice/peel, orange juice/peel, papaya, peas, peaches, persimmon


## Lutein

- Orange-red color.
- Often paired up with zeaxanthin, especially when it comes to the eyes.

**Possible Uses**
- Age-related macular degeneration[1314], Alzheimer's[1315], angina pectoris[1316], cataracts[1317], cardiovascular health[1318], cervical cancer, colon cancer[1319], colorectal cancer[1320], coronary artery disease[1321], diabetes eye health[1322], food coloring, glaucoma[1323], HIV[1324], infertility, lung cancer[1325], osteoarthritis, pancreatic cancer[1326], Parkinson's[1327], photophobia (light sensitivity)[1328], pneumonia, premenopausal breast cancer risk[1329], retinal health[1330], stomach cancer[1331]

**Properties**
- antioxidant, chemopreventive[1332]

**Food Sources**
- Synthasized only by plants.
- Broccoli, sprouts, carrots, celery, chicken fat and skin, collard greens, corn, *dandelion greens raw. egg yolk, garden peas, green leafy vegetables, *nasturtium leaves and *yellow flowers, *kale, kiwifruit, orange, orange pepper, pistachio nuts, romaine lettuce, spinach, squash, *Swiss chard, tomatoes, turnip greens, zucchini
- Sublingual spray

# Zeaxanthin

- Often paired up with lutein.

## Possible Uses
- Age-related macular degeneration[1333], Alzheimer's[1334], angina pectoris, asthma, atherosclerosis[1335], breast cancer[1336], cardiovascular health[1337], cataracts, cervical cancer, cataracts[1338], cervical dysplasia, dementia[1339], diabetic retinopathy[1340], eye problems, glaucoma[1341], HIV[1342], glaucoma[1343], lung cancer[1344], macular pigment level, male fertility, non-Hodgkin lymphoma, osteoarthritis, photophobia (light sensitivity)[1345], pneumonia, premenopausal breast cancer risk[1346], pre-term infant retinopathy[1347], retinal health[1348]

## Possible Benefits
- Drawn to eye fovea, lens and macula.
- Protects eye cells.
- Induces neuroblastoma cell apoptosis while not hurting healthy cells.[1349]
- Protects plants from excess energy that chlorophyll can't use.

## Properties
- Anti-inflammatory, anticancer, highly activity antioxidant , antitumor proliferation[1350]

## Warning, Precautions and Side Effects
- Works very gradually.
- Smokers should not take zeaxantin supplements, increases cancer risk.

**Food Sources**

> • Asparagus, broccoli, chicory greens, corn, egg yolk, fruits, kale, leafy green vegetables, lettuce, mustard greens, spinach, Swiss chard, turnip greens, watercress, yellow fruits and vegetables

# Lipids

## Different types of Lipids
- Beta sitosterol, campesterol and stigmasterol
- Phospholipids

## Hydrolysable Group
- Made up of neutral fats, oils, waxes, glycolipids, and phospholipids.

## Nonhydrolysable Group
- Made up of fat-soluble vitamins and steroids.

- Crosses the blood-brain barrier.
- Not water soluble.
- Composed of fatty acids and glycerol.
- Release large amounts of energy.

## Beta Sitosterol
## Beta Sitosterol  Glycoside

## Possible Uses
- Allergies, Alzheimer's[1351], arteriosclerotic heart disease[1352], asthma, autoimmune disorder[1353], benign prostatic hyperplasia[1354], boosts immune system, breast cancer[1355], bronchitis, cancer[1356], cardiovascular disease[1357], cholesterol control, chronic fatigue syndrome, colds[1358], colon cancer[1359], Crohn's, diabetes[1360], fibromyalgia[1361], flu[1362], gallstones, HIV/AIDS[1363], HIV infection[1364], hair loss, heart disease, hepatitis C[1365], immune system disease[1366], leukemia[1367], menopausal symptoms,

migraines, multiple sclerosis[1368], pneumonia[1369], prostate cancer[1370], prostate gland enlargement, psoriasis, rheumatoid arthritis, sexual function, sinusitis, stomach cancer[1371], tuberculosis[1372]

## Possible Benefits
- Inhibit cholesterol absorption.

## Properties
- Ameliorative, anti-inflammatory, anticancer, antineoplastic, antipyretic, immunomodulator

## Food Sources
- African plum tree, avocados, banana pepper, basil, buckwheat, butter, canola oil, cilantro leaves, corn oil, eggs, fava beans, fennel, flaxseed, grape leaves, green alga Tydemania, hawthorn, lemon grass, margarine, nuts, olive oil, peanuts, pomegranates, rice bran, Serrano pepper, South African star grass pygeum, soybean oil, soybeans, stinging nettle, vegetable oil, wheat germ

## Campesterol

- Chemical structure close to cholesterol.
- Anabolic steroid boldenone precursor.

## Possible Uses
- Alzheimer's[1373], atherosclerosis, breast cancer[1374], cardiovascular disease[1375], cartilage degradation[1376], cholesterol control, cognitive functioning, colon cancer[1377], coronary heart disease[1378], lung cancer[1379], neurodegenerative disorders, obesity[1380], Parkinson's, prostate cancer[1381]

## Properties

- Anti-inflammatory, antibacterial, anticancer[1382], apoptotic[1383], cytotoxicity[1384]

## Food Sources
- Avocados, banana, coffee, cucumber, dandelion, egg, grapefruit, lemongrass (citronella), margarine, mayonnaise, oats, onion, nuts, peppers, pomegranate, potato, rapeseed, Typhonium blumei, vegetable oils

## Stigmasterol

## Possible Uses
- Alzheimer's[1385], atherosclerosis[1386], breast cancer[1387], cardiovascular health[1388], cholesterol control, cold, colon cancer[1389], diabetes, flu, headache, heart disease, inflammation, osteoarthritis[1390], multiple sclerosis[1391], Parkinson's, prostate cancer[1392], rheumatism, skin health and permeability

## Properties
- Ameliorating, anti-inflammatory, anti-osteoarthritis[1393], antibacterial, antigenotoxic, antihypercholesterolemic, antihyperlipidemic, antimicrobial, antioxidant, antisnake venom[1394], antitumor, apoptotic, cytotoxicity, diuretic, hypoglycaemic

## Food Sources
- Buckwheat, calabar beans, cocoa beans, L. siceraria, legumes, M. barteri, margarine, nuts, parkia speciosa seeds, poppy seed, rapeseed, seeds, soy oil, soybean, pomegranate, unpasteurized milk, vegetable oil
- Sapindus sayonara L (Sapindaceae) for snakebites and ulcers.[1395]

# Phospholipids

- Major component in all cell membranes.
- Contain choline except sphingomyelin.
- Provides cellular structure and support.
- Helps biological functioning in intestines and lungs with water/air surfaces.
- Helps enzymes supply hormones or neurotransmitters.

## Different types of phospholipids
- Phosphatidic acid (phosphatidate) (PA), phosphatidylethanolamine (cephalin), phosphatidylcholine (lecithin), phosphatidylserine (PS), phosphoinositides, phosphosphingolipids

## Phosphatidic acid    Phosphatidate    (PA)
## Lysophosphatidic acid   (LPA)

- Water soluble.
- Precursor to other lipid biosynthesis.
- Simplest form.
- Signaling molecule, acidic but carries a negative charge.
- LPA is found in the saliva, induced cell growth in esophagus, mouth, and pharynx.[1396]

## Possible Uses
- Acid reflux, Alzheimer's[1397], atherosclerosis[1398], atherosclerotic plaque[1399], breast cancer[1400], cancer[1401], cardiovascular disease[1402], cognitive health, diarrhea, digestion, energy, fibrosis[1403], gastrointestinal disorders,

HIV[1404], heartburn, infertility[1405], inflammation[1406], lean body mass, neurodegenerative disorders[1407], neuropathic pain[1408], neuropsychiatric disorders[1409], ovarian cancer, prostatic adenocarcinoma[1410], reproductive disorders[1411], resistance weight training, stomach ulcers, stress reduction, wound healing (upper digestive organs)[1412]

## Possible Benefits

- Concerned with hormone and biotic stress responses.[1413]
- Stimulates growth factor not by eliciting $Ca^{2+}$ ionophore but by stimulating the intracellular release of it.[1414]
- Stimulates platelet formation by producing arachidonic acid.[1415]
- Stimulates cell proliferation.
- Critical role for myelin membrane biosynthesis.[1416]
- Binds to synucleins, may increase memory function.[1417]
- LPA receptors are a potent signaling molecule, with many targets and a wide range of effects.[1418]
- LPA has many affects on developmental, physiological and pathological processes.[1419]
- LPA aids in vascular development through angiogenesis, vascular maturation and vasculogenesis as well as the formation of the blood brain barrier.[1420]

## Food Sources

- Cabbage, egg yolk, lecithin, Mallotus japonicas (ulcers), soybean, protein whey

# Phosphatidylcholine (PC)    Lecithin

- Choline is a component.
- PC is used to make acetylcholine, which aids in the brain energy transference.

## Possible Uses
  - Alcohol-induced liver disease[1421], Alzheimer's[1422], anxiety, bipolar disorder (manic-depressive)[1423], cholesterol control, circulation problems, cirrhosis[1424], diabetes (type 2), eczema, fatty liver disease, Friedrich's ataxia[1425], gallbladder disease, gallstones, gastrointestinal problems, (almost all) hepatic disorders[1426], hepatitis A, B, C, Huntington's[1427], kidney dialysis[1428], liver disease[1429], liver fibrosis[1430], memory loss, neural tube defects (+folic acid)[1431], neuropsychiatric disorders, olfaction and taste[1432], Parkinson's[1433], premenstrual syndrome (PMS), pre-senile dementia[1434], schizophrenia[1435], tardive dyskinesia[1436], thyroid hormone stimulation, Tourette's syndrome[1437]

## Possible Benefits
  - Helps repair cell membranes.
  - Vital for healthy liver function.
  - Aid with people who have low levels of acetylcholine.
  - Injection or IV's are used for:
      - Chest pain, cholesterol deposits, cosmetic injections, fat embolism, fat plaque artery deposits, liver disease, non-cancerous fatty tumors
  - Breaks down fat and exports it from the liver.
  - Lowers homocysteine levels.
  - Important for fetal central nervous system, cognitive, cellular membrane development.

## Properties

- Anti-inflammatory

## Warning, Precautions and Side Effects

- Do not feed soy products to pre-adolescent children, not even soy infant formula.  More information on this topic in volume 2 of this same series, "Real Foods".

## Food Sources

- Beef liver, cereals, chicken, cotton seed, egg yolk, fish eggs, fish roe, krill oil, legumes, marine sources, milk, mustard, non-sticking cooking spray, nuts, organ meat, protein whey, rape seed, seed embryos, sheep brain, shrimp, soybean, squid, sunflower

## Research

There are about 80 Neural Tube Defects (NTD).  A study of 409 pregnancies were examined, in which, the women with lower choline experienced a higher risk and women with higher choline had lower risk for NTD.[1438]

FYI: NTD are birth defects that occur with an opening in the brain or in the spinal cord.
Anencephaly (without brain), ephalic disorder, cranium bifidum, schizencephaly, spina bifida

# Phosphatidylserine  (PS)
## Lysophosphatidylserine (LPS)

## Possible Uses
  - ADD/ADHD[1439], Alzheimer's[1440], cognitive improvement, cortisol blocker[1441], exercise-induced stress[1442], hormonal balance, memory, mental stress[1443], muscle soreness, neurodevelopment disorders, obesity[1444], Parkinson's[1445], scopolamine-induced amnesia[1446], senile dementia[1447], thyroid, weight training[1448]

## Possible Benefits
  - Many of the studies have been done with the therapeutic effects resulting from PS from cow's brains.
  - Enhances activation of bone marrow connective tissue mast cells.[1449]
  - Children with autism, in the erythrocyte membrane, have lower phosphatidylethanolamine (PE) and higher levels of phosphatidylserine (PS) levels than their siblings without autism.[1450]

## Food Sources
  - Anchovy, Atlantic cod, herring and mackerel, beef, *bovine brain (caution: mad cow disease transference), cabbage, chicken breast with skin, chicken heart and liver, crayfish, cuttlefish, eel, liver, mullet, pig kidney, *lamb kidney, liver and spleen, pork, soft-shell clam, *soy lecithin (thyroid inhibitor), trout, tuna, turkey, veal, white beans, whole grain barley

# FOOTNOTES


1 Dilip Ghosh and Tetsuya Konishi. "Anthocyanins and anthocyanin-rich extracts: role in diabetes and eye function" Asia Pac J Clin Nutr. 2007, vol 16(2), pp 200-208.

2 Dilip Ghosh and Tetsuya Konishi. "Anthocyanins and anthocyanin-rich extracts: role in diabetes and eye function" Asia Pac J Clin Nutr. 2007, vol 16(2), pp 200-208.

3 Hearn A and Bakri S. "Inhalable Composition." US Patent US 2010/0236562 A1. Date: Sep 23, 2020.

4 Frankic T, et al. "Use of Herbs and Spices and their Extracts in Animal Nutrition." Acta argiculturae Slovenica. 2009, vol 94(2), pp 95-102.

5 Ber A. "Neutralization of Phenolic (Aromatic) Food Compounds in a Holistic General Practice." Journal of Orthomolecular Psychiatry. 1984, pp 283-291.

6 Ibid.

7 Frankic T, et al. "Use of Herbs and Spices and their Extracts in Animal Nutrition." Acta argiculturae Slovenica. 2009, vol 94(2), pp 95-102.

8 Duke JA. "Handbook of Medicinal Herbs, Second Edition." CRC Press. Boca Raton. 2002. p. 555.

9 Ber A. "Neutralization of Phenolic (Aromatic) Food Compounds in a Holistic General Practice." Journal of Orthomolecular Psychiatry. 1984, pp 283-291.

10 Duke JA. "Handbook of Medicinal Herbs, Second Edition." CRC Press. Boca Raton. 2002. p. 555.

11 Ibid.

12 Moran AE, et al. "Carnosol Inhibits $\beta$-Catenin Tyrosine Phosphorylation and Prevents Adenoma Formation in the C57BL/6J/Min/+ (Min/+) Mouse." Cancer Res. 2005, vol 65, p 1097.

[13]   Fawcett JR, et al. "Inactivation of the human brain muscarinic acetylcholine receptor by oxidative damage catalyzed by a low molecular weight endogenous inhibitor from Alzheimer's brain is prevented by pyrophosphate analogs, bioflavonoids and other antioxidants." Brain Research. 2002, vol 950(1-2), pp 10-20.

[14]   Moran AE, et al. "Carnosol Inhibits β-Catenin Tyrosine Phosphorylation and Prevents Adenoma Formation in the C57BL/6J/Min/+ (Min/+) Mouse." Cancer Res. 2005, vol 65, p 1097.

[15]   Zunino SJ and Storms DH. Carnosol delays chemotherapy-induced DNA fragmentation and morphological changes associated with apoptosis in leukemic cells. Nutr Cancer. 2009, vol 61910, pp 94-102.

[16]   Kyota Fujita, et al. "Therapeutic Approach to Neurodegenerative Diseases by Medical Gases: Focusing on Redox Signaling and Related Antioxidant Enzymes." Oxidative Medicine and Cellular Longevity. 2012, Article ID 324256, 9 pagesdoi:10.1155/2012/324256.

[17]   Sinkovic A, et al. Rosemary extracts improve flow-mediated dilatation of the brachial artery and plasma PAI-1 activity in healthy young volunteers. Phytother Res. 2011, vol 25(3), pp 402-407.

[18]   Johnson JJ. "Carnosol: A promising anti-cancer and anti-inflammatory agent." Cancer Letters. 2011, vol 305(1), pp 1-7.

[19]   Ibid.

[20]   Moreno S, et al. "Antioxidant and antimicrobial activities of rosemary extracts linked to their polyphenol composition." Free Radical Research. 2006, vol 30(2), pp 223-231.

[21]   Kyota Fujita, et al. "Therapeutic Approach to Neurodegenerative Diseases by Medical Gases: Focusing on Redox Signaling and Related Antioxidant Enzymes." Oxidative Medicine and Cellular Longevity. 2012, Article ID 324256, 9 pagesdoi:10.1155/2012/324256.

[22]   Johnson JJ. "Carnosol: A promising anti-cancer and anti-inflammatory agent." Cancer Letters. 2011, vol 305(1), pp 1-7.

[23]  Chen CC, et al. Upregulation of NF-E2-related factor-2-dependent glutathione by carnosol provokes a cytoprotective response and enhances cell survival. Acta Pharmacol Sin. 2011, vol 32(1), pp 62-69.

[24]  Johnson JJ. "Carnosol: A promising anti-cancer and anti-inflammatory agent." Cancer Letters. 2011, vol 305(1), pp 1-7.

[25]  Fawcett JR, et al. "Inactivation of the human brain muscarinic acetylcholine receptor by oxidative damage catalyzed by a low molecular weight endogenous inhibitor from Alzheimer's brain is prevented by pyrophosphate analogs, bioflavonoids and other antioxidants." Brain Research. 2002, vol 950(1-2), pp 10-20.

[26]  Perry N, et al. "WHY SAGE MAY BE A WISE REMEDY: EFFECS OF SALVIA O THE NERVOUS SYSTEM." Overseas Publishers Association.  Harwood Academic Publishers.  2000,  pp 207-223.

[27]  Ferris-Tortajada J, et al. [Dietetic factors associated with prostate cancer: protective effects of Mediterranean diet]. Actas Urol Espl. 2012, vol 36(4), pp 239-245.

[28]  Johnson JJ. "Carnosol: A promising anti-cancer and anti-inflammatory agent." Cancer Letters. 2011, vol 305(1), pp 1-7.

[29]  Shirasuqi, et al. Novel screening method for potential skin-whitening compounds by a luciferase reporter assay. Biosci Biotechnol Biochem. 2010, vol 74(11), pp 2253-2258.

[30]  Sang Yong Kim, et al. "The Plant Phenolic Diterpene Carnosol Suppresses Sodium Nitroprusside-Induced Toxicity in C6 Glial Cells." J Agric Food Chem. 2010, vol 58(3), pp 1543-1550.

[31]  Ibid.

[32]  Johnson JJ. "Carnosol: A promising anti-cancer and anti-inflammatory agent." Cancer Letters. 2011, vol 305(1), pp 1-7.

[33]  Ibid.

[34]  Sang Yong Kim, et al. "The Plant Phenolic Diterpene Carnosol Suppresses Sodium Nitroprusside-Induced Toxicity in C6 Glial Cells." <u>J Agric Food Chem.</u> 2010, vol 58(3), pp 1543-1550.

[35]  Johnson JJ. "Carnosol: A promising anti-cancer and anti-inflammatory agent."

[36] Aruoma OI, et al. "Antioxidant and pro-oxidant properties of active rosemary constituents: carnosol and carnosic acid." 1991. Published online 22 Sep 2008. pp 257-268.
http://www.tandfonline.com/doi/abs/10.3109/00498259209046624

[37]  Ibid.

[38]  Ibid.

[39]  Johnson JJ. "Carnosol: A promising anti-cancer and anti-inflammatory agent."

[40]  Hearn A and Bakri S. "Inhalable Composition." US Patent US 2010/0236562 A1. Date: Sep 23, 2020.

[41]  Obaidat RM, et al. Preparation of mucoadhesive oral patches containing tetracycline hydrochloride and carvacrol for treatment of local mouth bacterial infections and candidiasis. Sci Pharm. 2011, vol 79(1), pp 197-212.

[42]  Ibid.

[43]  Obaidat RM, et al. Preparation of mucoadhesive oral patches containing tetracycline hydrochloride and carvacrol for treatment of local mouth bacterial infections and candidiasis. Sci Pharm. 2011, vol 79(1), pp 197-212.

[44]  Hotta M, et al. "Carvacrol, a component of thyme oil, activates PPARα and γ and suppresses COX-2 expression." <u>Journal of Lipid Research.</u> 2010, vol 51, pp 132-139.

[45]  Obaidat RM, et al. Preparation of mucoadhesive oral patches containing tetracycline hydrochloride and carvacrol for treatment of local mouth bacterial infections and candidiasis. Sci Pharm. 2011, vol 79(1), pp 197-212.

46  Hotta M, et al. "Carvacrol, a component of thyme oil, activates PPARα and γ and suppresses COX-2 expression." <u>Journal of Lipid Research.</u> 2010, vol 51, pp 132-139.

47  Kisko G and Roller S. "Carvacrol and *p*-cymene inactivate *Escherichia coli* O157:H7 in apple juice." <u>BMC microbiology.</u> 2005, vol 5, p 36.

48  Ananda Staff. Carvacrol Examined for anti-cancer effects on liver cells. Ananda Apothecary Forums.
Yin QH, et al. Anti-proliferative and pro-apoptotic effect of carvacrol on human hepatocellular carcinoma cell line HepG-2. Cytotechnology. 2011

49  Obaidat RM, et al. Preparation of mucoadhesive oral patches containing tetracycline hydrochloride and carvacrol for treatment of local mouth bacterial infections and candidiasis. Sci Pharm. 2011, vol 79(1), pp 197-212.

50  Can Baser KH. "Biological and Pharmacological Activities of Carvacrol and Carvacrol Bearing Essential Oils." <u>Current Pharmaceutical Design.</u> 2008, voll 14(29), pp 3106-3119.

51  "LIU Study: Component in Oregano kills Prostate Cancer Cells." BK PR Oregano & Cancer. Apr 25, 2012. Brooklyn NY.

52  Obaidat RM, et al. Preparation of mucoadhesive oral patches containing tetracycline hydrochloride and carvacrol for treatment of local mouth bacterial infections and candidiasis. Sci Pharm. 2011, vol 79(1), pp 197-212.

53  Ibid.

54  Hotta M, et al. "Carvacrol, a component of thyme oil, activates PPARα and γ and suppresses COX-2 expression." <u>Journal of Lipid Research.</u> 2010, vol 51, pp 132-139.

55  Can Baser KH. "Biological and Pharmacological Activities of Carvacrol and Carvacrol Bearing Essential Oils." <u>Current Pharmaceutical Design.</u> 2008, voll 14(29), pp 3106-3119.

56  Obaidat RM, et al. Preparation of mucoadhesive oral patches containing tetracycline hydrochloride and carvacrol for treatment of local mouth bacterial infections and candidiasis. Sci Pharm. 2011, vol 79(1), pp 197-212.

[57]  Can Baser KH. "Biological and Pharmacological Activities of Carvacrol and Carvacrol Bearing Essential Oils." Current Pharmaceutical Design. 2008, voll 14(29), pp 3106-3119.

[58]  Ibid.

[59]  Ibid.

[60]  Ibid.

[61]  Ibid.

[62]  Ibid.

[63]  Hearn A and Bakri S. "Inhalable Composition." US Patent US 2010/0236562 A1. Date: Sep 23, 2020.

[64]  Kaur GJ and Arora DS. "Bioactive potential of *Anethum graveolens*, *Foeniculum vulgare* and *Trachyspermum ammi* belonging to the family Umbelliferae - Current status." Journal of Medicinal Plants Research. 2010, vol 4(2), pp 087-094.

[65]  Ibid.

[66]  Ibid.

[67]  Abdallah HM and Ezzat SM. "Effect of the method of preparation on the composition and cytotoxic activity of the essential oil of Pituranthos tortuous." Z Naturforsch C. 2011, vol 66(3-4), pp 143-148.

[68]  Kaur GJ and Arora DS. "Bioactive potential of *Anethum graveolens*, *Foeniculum vulgare* and *Trachyspermum ammi* belonging to the family Umbelliferae - Current status." Journal of Medicinal Plants Research. 2010, vol 4(2), pp 087-094.

[69]  Nacim Zouari, et al. "Volatile and lipid analyses by gas chromatography/mass spectrometry and nutraceutical potential of edible wild Malva aegyptiaca L. (Malvaceae)." Int J of Food Sciences and Nutrition. 2011, vol 62(6), pp 600-608.

[70] Abdallah HM and Ezzat SM. "Effect of the method of preparation on the composition and cytotoxic activity of the essential oil of Pituranthos tortuous." Z Naturforsch C. 2011, vol 66(3-4), pp 143-148.

[71] Kaur GJ and Arora DS. "Bioactive potential of *Anethum graveolens*, *Foeniculum vulgare* and *Trachyspermum ammi* belonging to the family Umbelliferae - Current status." Journal of Medicinal Plants Research. 2010, vol 4(2), pp 087-094.

[72] Ibid.

[73] Abdallah HM and Ezzat SM. "Effect of the method of preparation on the composition and cytotoxic activity of the essential oil of Pituranthos tortuous." Z Naturforsch C. 2011, vol 66(3-4), pp 143-148.

[74] Omar S, et al. "Antimalarial activities of gedunin and 7-methoxygedunin and synergistic activity with dilation." Annals of Applied Biology. 2003, vol 143(2), pp 135-141.

[75] Kaur GJ and Arora DS. "Bioactive potential of *Anethum graveolens*, *Foeniculum vulgare* and *Trachyspermum ammi* belonging to the family Umbelliferae - Current status." Journal of Medicinal Plants Research. 2010, vol 4(2), pp 087-094.

[76] Ibid.

[77] Ibid.

[78] Ibid.

[79] Ibid.

[80] Ibid.

[81] Ibid.

[82] Ibid.

83    Ibid.


84    Parise_Filho, et al. "Dillapiole as Antileishmanial Agent: Discovery, Cytotoxic Activity and Preliminary SAR Studies of Dillapiole Analogues." <u>Archiv der Pharmazie</u>. 2012, vol 345(12), pp 934-944.


85    Omar S, et al. "Antimalarial activities of gedunin and 7-methoxygedunin and synergistic activity with dilation." <u>Annals of Applied Biology.</u> 2003, vol 143(2), pp 135-141.
86    Kaur GJ and Arora DS. "Bioactive potential of *Anethum graveolens*, *Foeniculum vulgare* and *Trachyspermum ammi* belonging to the family Umbelliferae - Current status." <u>Journal of Medicinal Plants Research.</u> 2010, vol 4(2), pp 087-094.


87    Loder JW, Moorhouse A, and Russell GB. "Tumour inhibitory plants. Amides of *Piper novae-hollandiae* (Piperaceae)." <u>Australian Journal of Chemistry.</u> 1969, vol 22(7), pp 1531-1538.


88    Kaur GJ and Arora DS. "Bioactive potential of *Anethum graveolens*, *Foeniculum vulgare* and *Trachyspermum ammi* belonging to the family Umbelliferae - Current status." <u>Journal of Medicinal Plants Research.</u> 2010, vol 4(2), pp 087-094.


89    Ibid.


90    Shabtay A, et al. "Synergistic antileukemic activity of carnosic acid-rich rosemary extract and the 19-nor Gemini vitamin D analogue in a mouse model of systemic acute myeloid leukemia." <u>Oncology</u>. 2008, vol 753-4, pp 203-214.


91    Hearn A and Bakri S. "Inhalable Composition." US Patent US 2010/0236562 A1. Date: Sep 23, 2020.


92    Warikoo R, et al. "Oviposition-altering and ovicidal potentials of five essential oils against female adults of the dengue vector, Aedes aegypti L." <u>Parasitol Res</u>. 2011, vol 109(4), pp 1125-1131.


93    Rand PW, et al. "Trial of a minimal-risk botanical compound to control the vector tick of Lyme disease." <u>J Med Entomol</u>. 2010, vol 47(4), pp 695-698.

94   Hearn A and Bakri S. "Inhalable Composition." US Patent US 2010/0236562 A1. Date: Sep 23, 2020.

95   Otang WM, et al. "Phytochemical studies and antioxidant activity of two South African medicinal plants traditionally used for the management of opportunistic fungal infections in HIV/AIDS patients." BMC Complementary and Alternative Medicine. 2012, vol 12, p 43.

96   Kelsey N, et al. "Neuroprotective effects of anthocyanins on apoptosis induced by mitochondrial oxidative stress." Nutritional Neuroscience. 2011, vol 14(6), pp 249-259(11).

97   Ibid.

98   Zafra-Stone S. et al. Berry anthocyanins as novel antioxidants in human health and disease prevention. Molecular Nutrition & Food Research. 2007, vol 51 (6), pp 675-683.

99   Wedick NM, et al. "Dietary flavonoid intakes and risk of type 2 diabetes in US men and women." Am J Clin Nutr. 2012, vol 95(4), pp 925-933.

100   Zafra-Stone S. et al. "Berry anthocyanins as novel antioxidants in human health and disease prevention." Molecular Nutrition & Food Research. 2007, vol 51 (6), pp 675-683.

101   Kelsey N, et al. "Neuroprotective effects of anthocyanins on apoptosis induced by mitochondrial oxidative stress." Nutritional Neuroscience. 2011, vol 14(6), pp 249-259(11).

102   Ibid.

103   Ibid.

104   Rasmussen SE, et al. "Dietary proanthocyanidins: Occurrence, dietary intake, bioavailability, and protection against cardiovascular disease." Molecular nutrition & Food Research. 2005, vol 49(2), pp 159-174.

105   Won-Ho Shin, Sang-Joon Park, and Eun-Joo Kim. "Protective effect of anthocyanins in middle cerebral artery occlusion and reperfusion model of cerebral ischemia in rats." Life Sciences. 2006, vol 79(2), pp 130-137.

[106]   Cvorovic J, et al. "Oxidative stress-based cytotoxicity of delphinidin and cyanidin in colon cancer cells." <u>Arch Biochem Biophys.</u> 2010, vol 50 (1), pp 151-157.

[107]   Sun CD, et al. "Cyanidin-3-glucoside-rich extract from Chinese bayberry fruit protects pancreatic B cells and ameliorates hyperglycemia in stretocin-induced diabetic mice." <u>J Med Food</u>. 2012, vol 15 (3), pp 288-298.

[108]   Palikova I, et al. "Constituents and antimicrobial properties of blue honeysuckle: a novel source for phenolic antioxidants." <u>J Agric Food Chem</u>. 2008, vol 56 (24), pp 11883-11889.

[109]   Ibid.

[110]   Guo H, et al. "Cyanidin-3-0-B-glucoside regulates fatty acid metabolism via an AMP-activated protein kinase-dependent signaling pathway in human HepG2 cells." <u>Lipids Health Dis.</u> 2012, vol 11, p 10.

[111]   Katsuzaki H, et al. "Cyanidin 3-O-beta-D-glucoside isolated from skin of black Glycine max and other anthocyanins isolated from skin of red grape induce apoptosis in human lymphoid leukemia Molt 4B cells." <u>Oncology Reports</u>. 2003, vol 10(2), pp 297-300.

[112]   Takanori T, et al. "Protective Effects of Dietary Cyanidin 3-$O$-$\beta$-d-Glucoside on Liver Ischemia–Reperfusion Injury in Rats." <u>Archives of Biochemistry and Biophysics.</u> 1999, vol 368(2), pp 361-366.

[113]   Pei-Ni Chen, et al. "Mulberry anthocyanins, cyanidin 3-rutinoside and cyanidin 3-glucoside, exhibited an inhibitory effect on the migration and invasion of a human lung cancer cell line." <u>Cancer Letters</u>. 2006, vol 235(2), pp 2480259.

[114]   Amorini AM, et al. "Cyanidin-3- O -$\beta$-glucopyranoside Protects Myocardium and Erythrocytes from Oxygen Radical-mediated Damages." <u>Free Radical Research.</u> 2003, vol 37(4), pp 453-460.

[115]   Prior RL, et al. "Whole Berries versus Berry Anthocyanins: Interactions with Dietary Fat Levels in the C57BL/6J Mouse Model of Obesity." <u>J Agric Food Chem.</u> 2008, vol 56(3), pp 647-653.

[116]   Munoz-Espada AC and Watkins BA. "Cyanidin attenuates $PGE_2$ production and cyclooxygenase-2 expression in LNCaP human prostate cancer cells." Journal of Nutritional Biochemistry. 2006, vol 17(9), pp 589-596.

[117]   Nasri S, et al. "Chronic cyanididn-3-glucoside administration improves short-term spatial recognition memory but not passive avoidance learning and memory in streptozotocin-diabetic rats." Phytother Res. 2012, vol 26 (8), pp 1205-1210.

[118]   Cimino F, et al. "Effect of Cyanidin-3-*O*-glucoside on UVB-Induced Response in Human Keratinocytes." J Agric Food Chem. 2006, vol 54(11), pp 4041-4047.

[119]   Palikova I, et al. "Constituents and antimicrobial properties of blue honeysuckle: a novel source for phenolic antioxidants." J Agric Food Chem. 2008, vol 56 (24), pp 11883-11889.

[120]   Ibid.

[121]   Ibid.

[122]  Tarozzi A, et al. "Neuroprotective effects of cyanidin 3-O-glucopyranoside on amyloid beta (25-35) oligomer-induced toxicity." Neurosci Lett. 2010, vol 473 (2), pp 72-76.

[123]  Hyo-Shin Kim, et al. "Delphinidin ameliorates beta-amyloid-induced neurotoxicity by inhibiting calcium influx and tar hyperphosphorylation." Bioscience, Biotechnology, and Biochemistry. 2009, vol 73(7), pp 1685-1689.

[124]   Martin S, et al. "Delphinidin, an active compound of red wine, inhibits endothelial cell apoptosis *via* nitric oxide pathway and regulation of calcium homeostasis." British Journal of Pharmacology. 2003, vol 139(6), pp 1095-1102.

[125]  Ozbay T and Nahta R.  "Delphinidin Inhibits HER2 and Erk½ Signaling and Suppresses Growth of HER2-Overexpressing and Triple Negative Breast Cancer Cell Lines." Breast Cancer. 2011, vol 5, pp 143-154.

[126]   Martin S, et al. "Delphinidin, an active compound of red wine, inhibits endothelial cell apoptosis *via* nitric oxide pathway and regulation of calcium homeostasis." British Journal of Pharmacology. 2003, vol 139(6), pp 1095-1102.

[127]  Cvorovic J, et al. "Oxidative stress-based cytotoxicity of delphinidin and cyaniding in colon cancer cells." <u>Arch Biochem Biophys.</u> 2010, vol 501 (1), pp 151-157.

[128]  Domitrovic R and Jakovac H. Antifibrotic activity of anthocyanidin delphinidin in carbon tetrachloride-induced hepatotoxicity. Toxicology. 2010, vol 272 (1-3), pp 1-10.

[129]  Dreiseitel A, et al. "Potential neuroprotective role of anthocyanins and anthocyanidins mediated by proteasome inhibition." <u>Pharmacopsychiatry.</u> 2007, vol 40, p A223.

[130]  Prior RL, et al. "Whole Berries versus Berry Anthocyanins: Interactions with Dietary Fat Levels in the C57BL/6J Mouse Model of Obesity." <u>J Agric Food Chem.</u> 2008, vol 56(3), pp 647-653.

[131]  X Gao, et al. "Habitual intake of dietary flavonoids and risk of Parkinson disease." <u>Neurology.</u> 2012, vol 78(15), pp 1138-1145.

[132]  Santos J, et al. Inhibition of host- and bacteria-derived proteinases by natural anthocyanins. J periodontal Res. 2011, vol 46 (5), pp 550-557.

[133]  Hafeez BB, et al. "A Dietary Anthocyanidin Delphinidin Induces Apoptosis of Human Prostate Cancer PC3 Cells *In vitro* and *In vivo*: Involvement of Nuclear Factor-?B Signaling." <u>Cancer Res</u>. 2008, vol 68, p 8564.

[134]  Matsunaga N, et al. "Bilberry and its main constituents have neuroprotective effects against retinal neuronal damage in vitro and in vivo." <u>Molecular Nutrition & Food Research.</u> 2009, vol 53(7), pp 869-877.

[135]  Rodrigues AD, et al. "Neuroprotective and anticonvulsant effects of organic and conventional purple grape juices on seizures in Wistar rats induced by pentylenetetrazole." <u>neurochemistry International.</u> 2012, vol 60(8), pp 799-805.

[136]  Dreiseitel A, et al. "Potential neuroprotective role of anthocyanins and anthocyanidins mediated by proteasome inhibition." <u>Pharmacopsychiatry.</u> 2007, vol 40, p A223.

[137]  Afaq R and Katiyar SK. "Polyphenols: Skin Photoprotection and Inhibition of Photocarcinogenesis." <u>Mini Rev Med Chem.</u> 2011, vol 11 (14), pp 1200-1215.

138   Martin S, et al. "Delphinidin, an active compound of red wine, inhibits endothelial cell apoptosis *via* nitric oxide pathway and regulation of calcium homeostasis." British Journal of Pharmacology. 2003, vol 139(6), pp 1095-1102.

139   Sylvie L, et al. "Delphinidin, a dietary anthocyanidin, inhibits vascular endothelial growth factor receptor-2 phosphorylation." Carcinogenesis. 2006, vol 27(5), pp 989-996.

140   Clere N, et al. "Anticancer properties of falconoid: roles in various stages of carcinogenesis." Cardiovasc Hematol Agents Med Chem. 2001, vol 9 (2), pp 62-77.

141   Domitrovic R and Jakovac H. "Antifibrotic activity of anthocyanidin delphinidin in carbon tetrachloride-induced hepatotoxicity." Toxicology. 2010, vol 272 (1-3), pp 1-10.

142   Paixao J, et al. "Dietary anthocyanins protect endothelial cells against peroxynitrite-induced mitochondrial apoptosis pathway and Bax nuclear translocation: an in vitro approach." Apoptosis. 2011, vol 16 (10), pp 976-989.

143   Matsunaga N, et al. "Bilberry and its main constituents have neuroprotective effects against retinal neuronal damage in vitro and in vivo." Molecular Nutrition & Food Research. 2009, vol 53(7), pp 869-877.

144   Riviere C, et al. "New polyphenols active on $\beta$-amyloid aggregation." Bioorganic & Medicinal Chemistry Letters. 2008, vol 18(2), pp 828-831.

145   Liya Li, et al. *"Eugenia jambolana* Lam. Berry Extract Inhibits Growth and Induces Apoptosis of Human Breast Cancer but Not Non-Tumorigenic Breast Cells." J Agric Food Chem. 2009, vol 57(3), pp 826-231.

146   Persson IA, et al. a'Effect of Vaccinium myrtillus and its polyphenols on angiotensin converting enzyme activity in human endothelial cells." J Agric Food Chem. 2009, vol 10 (57), pp 4626-4629.

147   Wang Q, et al. "Inhibitory effect of antioxidant extracts from various potatoes on the proliferation of human colon and liver cancer cells." Nutr Cancer. 2011, vol 63 (7), pp 1044-1052.

[148]  Thomasset S, et al. "Pilot Study of Oral Anthocyanins for Colorectal Cancer Chemoprevention." <u>Cancer Prev Res.</u> 2009, vol 2, p 625.

[149]  Dilip Ghosh and Tetsuya Konishi. "Anthocyanins and anthocyanin-rich extracts: role in
diabetes and eye function" <u>Asia Pac J Clin Nutr.</u> 2007, vol 16(2), pp 200-208.

[150]  Ibid.

[151]  Shih PH, et al. "Effects of anthocyanidin on the inhibition of proliferation and induction of apoptosis in human gastric adenocarcinoma cells." <u>Food Chem Toxicol.</u> 2005, vol 43 (10), pp 1557-1566.

[152]  Katsube N, et al. Induction of apoptosis in cancer cells by Bilberry (Vaccinium myrtillus) and the anthocyanins. J Agric Food Chem. 2003, vol 51 (1), pp 68-75.

[153]  Wang Q, et al. Inhibitory effect of antioxidant extracts from various potatoes on the proliferation of human colon and liver cancer cells. Nutr Cancer. 2011, vol 63 (7), pp 1044-1052.

[154]  Riviere C, et al. "New polyphenols active on β-amyloid aggregation." <u>Bioorganic & Medicinal Chemistry Letters.</u> 2008, vol 18(2), pp 828-831.

[155]  Prior RL, et al. "Whole Berries versus Berry Anthocyanins: Interactions with Dietary Fat Levels in the C57BL/6J Mouse Model of Obesity." <u>J Agric Food Chem.</u> 2008, vol 56(3), pp 647-653.

[156]  X Gao, et al. "Habitual intake of dietary flavonoids and risk of Parkinson disease." <u>Neurology.</u> 2012, vol 78(15), pp 1138-1145.

[157]  Reddivari L, et al. "Anthocyanin fraction from potato extracts is cytotoxic to prostate cancer cells through activation of caspase-dependent and caspase-independent pathways." <u>Carcinogenesis.</u> 2007, vol 28(10), pp 2227-2235.

[158]  Pirker KF, et al. "Antiradical properties of red wine portisins." <u>J Agric Food Chem.</u> 2001, vol59 (21), pp 11833-11837.

[159]  Matsunaga N, et al. "Bilberry and its main constituents have neuroprotective effects against retinal neuronal damage in vitro and in vivo." <u>Mol Nutr Food Res.</u> 2009, vol 53 (7), pp 869-877.

[160]   Wang Q, et al. Inhibitory effect of antioxidant extracts from various potatoes on the proliferation of human colon and liver cancer cells. Nutr Cancer. 2011, vol 63 (7), pp 1044-1052.

[161]   Pirker KF, et al. Antiradical properties of red wine portisins. J Agric Food Chem. 2001, vol59 (21), pp 11833-11837.

[162]   Hartman RE, et al. "Pomegranate juice decreases amyloid load and improves behavior in a mouse model of Alzheimer's disease." Neurobiology of Disease. 2006, vol 24(3), pp 506-515.

[163]   Moumita Roy, et al. "Action of pelargonidin on hyperglycemia and oxidative damage in diabetic rats: Implication for glycation-induced hemoglobin modification." Life Sciences. 2008, vol 82(21-22), pp 11102-1110.

[164]   Liya Li, et al. "*Eugenia jambolana* Lam. Berry Extract Inhibits Growth and Induces Apoptosis of Human Breast Cancer but Not Non-Tumorigenic Breast Cells." J Agric Food Chem. 2009, vol 57(3), pp 826-231.

[165]   Yasuko Noda, et al. "Antioxidant Activities of Pomegranate Fruit Extract and Its Anthocyanidins: Delphinidin, Cyanidin, and Pelargonidin." J Agric Food Chem. 2002, vol 50(1), pp 166-171.

[166]   Wang Q, et al. Inhibitory effect of antioxidant extracts from various potatoes on the proliferation of human colon and liver cancer cells. Nutr Cancer. 2011, vol 63 (7), pp 1044-1052.

[167]   Moumita Roy, et al. "Action of pelargonidin on hyperglycemia and oxidative damage in diabetic rats: Implication for glycation-induced hemoglobin modification." Life Sciences. 2008, vol 82(21-22), pp 11102-1110.

[168]   Roghani M, et al. Oral pelargonidin exerts dose-dependent neuroprotection in 6-hydroxydopamine rat model of hemi-parkinsonism. Brain Res Bull. 2010, vol 82 (5-6), pp 279-283.

[169]   Shin DY, et al. Induction of apoptosis and inhibition of invasion in human hepatoma cells by anthocyanins from meoru. Ann N Y Acad Sci. 2009, vol 1171, pp 137-148.

170  Kamenickova A, et al. "Pelargonidin activates the AhR and induces CYP1A1 in primary human hepatocytes and human cancer cell lines HepG2 and LS174T." Toxicology Letters. 2013, vol 218(3), pp 253-259.

171  Wang Q, et al. Inhibitory effect of antioxidant extracts from various potatoes on the proliferation of human colon and liver cancer cells. Nutr Cancer. 2011, vol 63 (7), pp 1044-1052.

172  Prior RL, et al. "Whole Berries versus Berry Anthocyanins: Interactions with Dietary Fat Levels in the C57BL/6J Mouse Model of Obesity." J Agric Food Chem. 2008, vol 56(3), pp 647-653.

173  Mirshekar M, et al. Chronic oral pelargonidin alleviates streptozotocin-induced diabetic neuropathic hyperalgesia in rat: involvement of oxidative stress. Iran Biomed J. 2010, vol 14 (1-2), pp 33-39.

174  Bhoopat L, et al. Hepatoprotective effects of lychee (Litchi chinensis Sonn.): a combination of antioxidant and anti-apoptotic activities. J Ethnopharmacol. 2011, vol 136 (1), pp 55-66.

175  Cesoniene L, et al. Phenolics and anthocyanins in berries of European cranberry and their antimicrobial activity. Medicina (Kaunas). 2009, vol 45 (12), pp 992-999.

176  Liya Li, et al. "*Eugenia jambolana* Lam. Berry Extract Inhibits Growth and Induces Apoptosis of Human Breast Cancer but Not Non-Tumorigenic Breast Cells." J Agric Food Chem. 2009, vol 57(3), pp 826-231.

177  Abdel-Moemin AR. Switching to black rice diets modulates low-density lipoprotein oxidation and lipid measurements in rabbits. Am J Med Sci. 2011, vol 341 (4), pp 318-324.

178  Poulose SM, et al. Anthocyanin-rich açai (Euterpe oleracea Mart.) fruit pulp fractions attenuate inflammatory stress signaling in mouse brain BV-2 microglial cells. J Agric Food Chem. 2012, vol 60 (4), pp 1084-1093.

179  Cuiwei Zhao, et al. "Effects of Commercial Anthocyanin-Rich Extracts on Colonic Cancer and Nontumorigenic Colonic Cell Growth." J Agric Food Chem. 2004, vol 52(20), pp 6122-6128.

180   Cesoniene L, et al. Phenolics and anthocyanins in berries of European cranberry and their antimicrobial activity. Medicina (Kaunas). 2009, vol 45 (12), pp 992-999.

181   Ibid.

182   Pei-Ni Chen, et al. "Cyanidin 3-Glucoside and Peonidin 3-Glucoside Inhibit Tumor Cell Growth and Induce Apoptosis In Vitro and Suppress Tumor Growth In Vivo." Nutrition and Cancer. 2005, vol 53(2), pp 232-243.

183   Ho ML, et al. "Peonidin 3-glucoside inhibits lung cancer metastasis by downregulation of proteinases activities and MAPK pathway." Nutr Cancer. 2010, vol 62 (4), pp 505-516.

184   Poulose SM, et al. "Anthocyanin-rich açai (Euterpe oleracea Mart.) fruit pulp fractions attenuate inflammatory stress signaling in mouse brain BV-2 microglial cells." J Agric Food Chem. 2012, vol 60 (4), pp 1084-1093.

185   Prior RL, et al. "Whole Berries versus Berry Anthocyanins: Interactions with Dietary Fat Levels in the C57BL/6J Mouse Model of Obesity." J Agric Food Chem. 2008, vol 56(3), pp 647-653.

186   Cesoniene L, et al. "Phenolics and anthocyanins in berries of European cranberry and their antimicrobial activity." Medicina (Kaunas). 2009, vol 45 (12), pp 992-999.

187   Ibid.

188   Abdel-Moemin AR. Switching to black rice diets modulates low-density lipoprotein oxidation and lipid measurements in rabbits. Am J Med Sci. 2011, vol 341 (4), pp 318-324.

189   Cesoniene L, et al. "Phenolics and anthocyanins in berries of European cranberry and their antimicrobial activity." Medicina (Kaunas). 2009, vol 45 (12), pp 992-999.

190   Li L, et al. "Eugenia jambolana Lam. berry extract inhibits growth and induces apoptosis of human breast cancer but not non-tumorigenic breast cells." J Agric Food Chem. 2009, vol 57 (3), pp 826-831.

[191]  Ibid.

[192]  Cesoniene L, et al. "Phenolics and anthocyanins in berries of European cranberry and their antimicrobial activity." <u>Medicina (Kaunas).</u> 2009, vol 45 (12), pp 992-999.

[193]  Li L, et al. "Eugenia jambolana Lam. berry extract inhibits growth and induces apoptosis of human breast cancer but not non-tumorigenic breast cells." <u>J Agric Food Chem.</u> 2009, vol 57(3), pp 826-831.

[194]  Arpita Basu, et al. "Berries: emerging impact on cardiovascular health." <u>Nutrition Reviews</u>. 20210, vol 68(3), pp 168-177.

[195]  Zu XY, et al. "Anthocyanins extracted from Chinese blueberry (Vaccinium uliginosum L.) and its anticancer effects on DLD-1 and COLO205 cells." <u>Chin Med J</u>. 2010, vol 123 (19), pp 271 4-2719.

[196]  Ibid.

[197]  You Q, et al. "Inhibitory effects of muscadine anthocyanins on $\alpha$-glucosidase and pancreatic lipase activities." <u>J Agric Food Chem.</u> 2011, vol 59 (17), pp 9506-9511.

[198]  Saito T, et al. "Anthocyanins from new red leaf tea 'Sunrouge'." <u>J Agric Food Chem</u>. 2011, vol 59 (9), pp 4779-4782.

[199]  Shin DY, et al. "Induction of apoptosis and inhibition of invasion in human hepatoma cells by anthocyanins from meoru." <u>Ann N Y Acad Sci</u>. 2009, vol1171, pp 137-148.

[200]  Ibid.

[201]  Prior RL, et al. "Whole Berries versus Berry Anthocyanins: Interactions with Dietary Fat Levels in the C57BL/6J Mouse Model of Obesity." <u>J Agric Food Chem.</u> 2008, vol 56(3), pp 647-653.

[202]  Matchett MD, et al. "Blueberry flavonoids inhibit matrix metalloproteinase activity in DU145 human prostate cancer cells." <u>Biochemistry and Cell Biology</u>. 2005, vol 83(5), pp 627-643.

203   Zu XY, et al. Anthocyanins extracted from Chinese blueberry (Vaccinium uliginosum L.) and its anticancer effects on DLD-1 and COLO205 cells. Chin Med J. 2010, vol 123 (19), pp 271 4-2719.

204   Shin DY, et al. "Induction of apoptosis and inhibition of invasion in human hepatoma cells by anthocyanins from meoru." Ann N Y Acad Sci. 2009, vol1171, pp 137-148.

205   Ibid.

206   Saito T, et al. Anthocyanins from new red leaf tea 'Sunrouge'. J Agric Food Chem. 2011, vol 59 (9), pp 4779-4782.
http://www.ncbi.nlm.nih.gov/pubmed/21480597

207   I Ibid.

208   Zu XY, et al. Anthocyanins extracted from Chinese blueberry (Vaccinium uliginosum L.) and its anticancer effects on DLD-1 and COLO205 cells. Chin Med J. 2010, vol 123 (19), pp 271 4-2719.

209   Kelly GE and Joannou GE. "Therapeutic Methods and Compositions Involving Isoflavones." US Patent. US2006/0286250 A1. Date: Dec 21, 2006.

210   Ibid.

211   Ibid.

212   Ibid.

213   Ibid.

214   Ibid.

215   Ibid.

216   Ibid.

217   Ibid.

[218]  Ibid.

[219]  Ibid.

[220]  Ibid.

[221]  Ibid.

[222]  Ibid.

[223]  Ibid.

[224]  Ibid.

[225]  Ibid.

[226]  Ibid.

[227]  Sosic-Jurjevic B, et al. "Suppressive effects of genistein and daidzein on pituitary-thyroid axis in orchidectomized middle-aged rats." Exp Biol Med (Maywood). 2010, vol 235(5), pp 590-598.

[228]  METHOD FOR THE INHIBITION OF ALDH-I USEFUL IN THE TREATMENT OF ALCOHOL DEPENDENCE OR ALCOHOL ABUSE.  European Patent EP0592583.

[229]  Clarkson TB, et al. "Methods for Inhibiting the Development of Alzheimer's Disease and Related Dementias and for Preserving Cognitive Function" US Patent #5,952,374, dated Sep. 14, 1999,

[230]  Pan W, et al. "Genistein, Daidzein and Glycitein Inhibit Growth and DNA Synthesis of Aortic Smooth Muscle Cells from Stroke-Prone Spontaneously Hypertensive Rats." J Nutr. 2001, vol 131(4), pp 1154-1158.

[231]  Ying Hua Gao and Masayoshi Yamaguchi. Anabolic effect of daidzein on cortical bone in tissue culture: Comparison with genistein effect. Molecular and Cellular Biochemistry. 1999, vol 194 (1-2), pp 93-98.

[232]  Wu AH, et al. Tofu and risk of breast cancer in Asian-Americans. Cancer Epidemiol Biomarkers Prev. 1996, vol 5, p 901.

233   Han KK, et al. "Benefits of Soy Isoflavone Therapeutic Regimen on Menopausal Symptoms." <u>Obstetrics & Gynecology.</u> 2002, vol 99(3),pp 389-394.

234   Clarkson TB, et al. "Methods for Inhibiting the Development of Alzheimer's Disease and Related Dementias and for Preserving Cognitive Function" US Patent #5,952,374, dated Sep. 14, 1999,

235   Ibid.

236   Ivan Palomo, et al. "Soybean Products Consumption in the Prevention of Cardiovascular Diseases." Soybean and Health.
www.intechopen.com
http://cdn.intechweb.org/pdfs/19741.pdf

237   Ollberding NJ, et al. Legume, soy, tofu, and isoflavone intake and endometrial cancer risk in postmenopausal women in the multiethnic cohort study. J Natl Cancer Inst. 2012, vol 104 (1), pp 67-76.

238   Pan W, et al. "Genistein, Daidzein and Glycitein Inhibit Growth and DNA Synthesis of Aortic Smooth Muscle Cells from Stroke-Prone Spontaneously Hypertensive Rats." <u>J Nutr.</u> 2001, vol 131(4), pp 1154-1158.

239   Ying Hua Gao and Masayoshi Yamaguchi. Anabolic effect of daidzein on cortical bone in tissue culture: Comparison with genistein effect. Molecular and Cellular Biochemistry. 1999, vol 194 (1-2), pp 93-98.

240   Han KK, et al. "Benefits of Soy Isoflavone Therapeutic Regimen on Menopausal Symptoms." <u>Obstetrics & Gynecology.</u> 2002, vol 99(3),pp 389-394.

241   Ivan Palomo, et al. "Soybean Products Consumption in the Prevention of Cardiovascular Diseases." Soybean and Health.
www.intechopen.com
http://cdn.intechweb.org/pdfs/19741.pdf

242   Ying Hua Gao and Masayoshi Yamaguchi. Anabolic effect of daidzein on cortical bone in tissue culture: Comparison with genistein effect. Molecular and Cellular Biochemistry. 1999, vol 194 (1-2), pp 93-98.

243   Singh-Gupta V, et al. "Daidzein effect on hormone refractory prostate cancer in vitro and in vivo compared to genistein and soy extract: potentiation of radiotherapy." <u>Pharm Res</u>. 2010, vol 27 (6), pp 1115-1127.

244   Mitsuru More, et al. "Traditional Japanese diet and prostate cancer." <u>Molecular Nutrition & Food Research</u>. 2009, vol 53 (2), pp 191-200.

245   Pan W, et al. "Genistein, Daidzein and Glycitein Inhibit Growth and DNA Synthesis of Aortic Smooth Muscle Cells from Stroke-Prone Spontaneously Hypertensive Rats." <u>J Nutr.</u> 2001, vol 131(4), pp 1154-1158.

246   Sharma S, et al. Ameliorative effect of daidzein: a caveolin-1 inhibitor in vascular endothelium dysfunction induced by ovariectomy. Indian J Exp Biol. 2012, vol 50 (1), pp 28-34.

247   Ivan Palomo, et al. "Soybean Products Consumption in the Prevention of Cardiovascular Diseases." Soybean and Health.

248   Wang H, et al. "[Study on HPLC chromatographic fingerprint of anti-tumor active site SSCE of Caulis spatholobi]." <u>Zhongguo Zhong Yao Za Zhi.</u> 2011, vol 36 (18), pp 2525-2529.

249   Janice Barlow, Jo Ann Johnson, and Lacie Scofield. "Early Life Exposure to the Phytoestrogen  and Daidzein Breast Cancer Risk in Later Years. FACT SHEET on the PHYTOESTROGEN Daidzein. **BCERC COTC Fact** Sheet – Phytoestrogen Genistein," BREAST CANCER & THE ENVIRONMENT RESEARCH CENTERS. 11/07/07

250   Maryam Bagherii. "Neuroprotective Effect of Genistein: Studies in Rat Models of Parkinson's and Alzheimer's Disease." Doctoral thesis, comprehensive summary. DiVA Academic Archives Online. <u>Linköping University Electronic Press</u>. 2012

251   Pan W, et al. "Genistein, Daidzein and Glycitein Inhibit Growth and DNA Synthesis of Aortic Smooth Muscle Cells from Stroke-Prone Spontaneously Hypertensive Rats." <u>J Nutr.</u> 2001, vol 131(4), pp 1154-1158.

252   Messing E, et al. "A phase 2 cancer chemoprevention biomarker trial of isoflavone G-2535 (genistein) in presurgical bladder cancer patients." <u>Cancer Prev Res</u>. 2012, vol 5 (4), pp 621-630.
http://www.ncbi.nlm.nih.gov/pubmed/22293631

253   Ghiringhelli F, et al. "Immunomodulation and anti-inflammatory roles of polyphenols as anticancer agents." <u>Anticancer Agents Med Chem</u>. 2012, vol 12 (8), pp 852-873.

254   Balabhadrapathruni S et al. "Effects of genistein and structurally related phytoestrogens on cell cycle kinetics and apoptosis in MDA-MB-468 human breast cancer cells." <u>Oncology Reports.</u> 2000, vol 7 (1), pp 3-12.

255   Dixon RA and Ferreira D.  "Genistein." <u>Phytochemistry.</u> 2002, vol 60(3), pp 205-211.

256   Banerjee S, et al. "Multi-targeted therapy of cancer by genistein." <u>Cancer Letters.</u> 2008, vol 269(2), pp 226-242.

257   Clarkson TB, et al. "Methods for Inhibiting the Development of Alzheimer's Disease and Related Dementias and for Preserving Cognitive Function" US Patent #5,952,374, dated Sep. 14, 1999,

258   Rao CV, et al. "Enhancement of Experimental Colon Cancer by Genistein." <u>Cancer Research.</u> 1997, vol 57,p3717.

259   Clarkson TB, et al. "Methods for Inhibiting the Development of Alzheimer's Disease and Related Dementias and for Preserving Cognitive Function" US Patent #5,952,374, dated Sep. 14, 1999,

260   Fu Z, et al. "Genistein induces pancreatic beta-cell proliferation through activation of multiple signaling pathways and prevents insulin-deficient diabetes in mice." <u>Endocrinology.</u>  2010, vol 151(7), pp 3026-3037.

261   Banerjee S, et al. "Multi-targeted therapy of cancer by genistein." <u>Cancer Letters.</u> 2008, vol 269(2), pp 226-242.

262   Pan W, et al. "Genistein, Daidzein and Glycitein Inhibit Growth and DNA Synthesis of Aortic Smooth Muscle Cells from Stroke-Prone Spontaneously Hypertensive Rats." <u>J Nutr.</u> 2001, vol 131(4), pp 1154-1158.

263   Lian F, et al. "Genistein-induced G2-m arrest, P21$^{WAF1}$ upregulation, and apoptosis in a non-small-cell lung cancer cell line." <u>Nutrition and Cancer.</u> 1998, vol 31(3), pp 184-191.

264   Haitao Luo et al. Inhibition of Cell Growth and VEGF Expression in Ovarian Cancer Cells by Flavonoids." <u>Nutrition and Cancer.</u> 2008, vol 60 (6).

265   Maryam Bagherii. "Neuroprotective Effect of Genistein: Studies in Rat Models of Parkinson's and Alzheimer's Disease." Doctoral thesis, comprehensive summary. DiVA Academic Archives Online. <u>Linköping University Electronic Press.</u> 2012

266   Dixon RA and Ferreira D.  "Genistein." <u>Phytochemistry.</u> 2002, vol 60(3), pp 205-211.

267   Ghiringhelli F, et al. Immunomodulation and anti-inflammatory roles of polyphenols as anticancer agents. Anticancer Agents Med Chem. 2012, vol 12 (8), pp 852-873.

268   Park CE, et al. The antioxidant effects of genistein are associated with AMP-activated protein kinase activation and PTEN induction in prostate cancer cells. J Med Food. 2010, vol 13 (4), pp 815-820.

269   Pan W, et al. "Genistein, Daidzein and Glycitein Inhibit Growth and DNA Synthesis of Aortic Smooth Muscle Cells from Stroke-Prone Spontaneously Hypertensive Rats." <u>J Nutr.</u> 2001, vol 131(4), pp 1154-1158.

270   Dixon RA and Ferreira D.  "Genistein." <u>Phytochemistry.</u> 2002, vol 60(3), pp 205-211.

271   Ghiringhelli F, et al. Immunomodulation and anti-inflammatory roles of polyphenols as anticancer agents. Anticancer Agents Med Chem. 2012, vol 12 (8), pp 852-873.

272   Ibid.

273   Ibid.

274   Ma W, et al. Genistein as a neuroprotective antioxidant attenuates redox imbalance induced by beta-amyloid peptides 25-35 in PC12 cells. Int J Dev Neurosci. 2010, vol 28 (4), pp 289-295.

275   Janice Barlow, Jo Ann Johnson, and Lacie Scofield. Early Life Exposure to the Phytoestrogen Genistein and Breast Cancer Risk in Later Years. FACT SHEET on the PHYTOESTROGEN GENISTEIN. BCERC COTC Fact Sheet – Phytoestrogen Genistein, BREAST CANCER & THE ENVIRONMENT RESEARCH CENTERS. 11/07/07

276   Ibid.

277   Haitao Luo et al.  Inhibition of Cell Growth and VEGF Expression in Ovarian Cancer Cells by Flavonoids. Nutrition and Cancer. 2008, vol 60 (6).

278   Pan W, et al. "Genistein, Daidzein and Glycitein Inhibit Growth and DNA Synthesis of Aortic Smooth Muscle Cells from Stroke-Prone Spontaneously Hypertensive Rats." J Nutr. 2001, vol 131(4),, pp 1154-1158.

279   Wu AH, et al. "Epidemiology of soy exposures and breast cancer risk." British Journal of Cancer. 2008, vol 98, pp 9-14.

280   Pan W, et al. "Genistein, Daidzein and Glycitein Inhibit Growth and DNA Synthesis of Aortic Smooth Muscle Cells from Stroke-Prone Spontaneously Hypertensive Rats." J Nutr. 2001, vol 131(4),, pp 1154-1158.

281   Xiao JX, et al. Soy-derived isoflavones inhibit HeLa cell growth by inducing apoptosis. Plant Foods Hum Nutr. 2011, vol 66 (2), pp 122-128.

282   Bielecki A, et al. Estrogen receptor-$\beta$ mediates the inhibition of DLD-1 human colon adenocarcinoma cells by soy isoflavones. Nutr Cancer. 2011, vol 63 (1), 139-150.

283   Toyomura K, et al. "Soybeans, Soy Foods, Isoflavones and Risk of Colorectal Cancer: a Review of Experimental and Epidemiological Data." Asian Pacific J Cancer Prev. 2002, vol 3, pp 125-132.

284   Bhathena SJ and Velasquez MT. "Beneficial role of dietary phytoestrogens in obesity and diabetes." Am J Clin Nutr. 2002, vol 76(6), PP 1191-1201.

[285]   Ollberding NJ,et al. Legume, soy, tofu, and isoflavone intake and endometrial cancer risk in postmenopausal women in the multiethnic cohort study. J Natl Cancer Inst. 2012, vol 104 (1), pp 67-76.

[286]   Noel J-C, et al. "Ureteral mullerian carcinosarcoma (mixed mullerian tumor) associated with endometriosis occurring in a patient with a concentrated soy isoflavones supplementation." Archives of Gynecology and Obstetrics. 2006, vol 274(6), pp 389-392.

[287]   Bhathena SJ and Velasquez MT. "Beneficial role of dietary phytoestrogens in obesity and diabetes." Am J Clin Nutr. 2002, vol 76(6), PP 1191-1201.

[288]   Bandera EV, et al. Phytoestrogen consumption from foods and supplements and epithelial ovarian cancer risk: a population-based case control study. BMC Womens Health. 2011, vol 23, p 40.

[289]   Clubbs EA and Bomser JA. Basal cell induced differentiation of noncancerous prostate epithelial cells (RWPE-1) by glycitein. Nutr Cancer. 2009, vol 61 (3), pp 390-396.

[290]   Pan W, et al. "Genistein, Daidzein and Glycitein Inhibit Growth and DNA Synthesis of Aortic Smooth Muscle Cells from Stroke-Prone Spontaneously Hypertensive Rats." J Nutr. 2001, vol 131(4),, pp 1154-1158.

[291]   Pyo YH and Seong KS. "Hypolipidemic effects of Monascus-fermented soybean extracts in rats fed a high-fat and -cholesterol diet." J Agric Food Chem. 2009, vol 57 (18), pp 8617-8622.

[292]  Romero-Matos G. "Devastating treatment against HIV/AIDS with Capsaicin." US Patent. US2004/0224037 A1. Date: Nov 11, 2004.

[293]    Jih-Pyang Wang et al.  "Antithemostatic and antthrombotic effects of capsaicin in comparison with aspirin and indomethacin."  Thrombosis Research. 1985, vol 37 (6) pp 669-679

[294]   C. Peter and N Watson. "Topical capsaicin as an adjuvant analgesic." Journal of Pain and Symptom Management. 1994, vol 9(7), pp 425-433.

[295]   Deal CL, et al "Treatment of arthritis with topical capsaicin: a double-blind trial." Clinical Therapeutics. 1991, vol 13(3), pp 383-395.

[296]  Szallasi A. "Vanilloid (Capsaicin) Receptors in Health and Disease." AJCP. 2002, vol 118, pp 110-121.

[297]  Vaishnava P and Wang DH. "Capsaicin Sensitive-Sensory Nerves and Blood Pressure Regulation." Current Medicinal Chemistry - Cardiovascular & Hematological Agents. 2003, vol 1(2), pp 177-188(12).

[298]  Ghilardi JR, et al. "Selective Blockade of the Capsaicin Receptor TRPV1 Attenuates Bone Cancer Pain." Journal of Neuroscience. 2005, vol 25(12), pp 3126-3131.

[299]  Thoennissen NH, et al. "Capsaicin causes cell-cycle arrest and apoptosis in *ER*-positive and -negative breast cancer cells by modulating the *EGFR/HER-2* pathway." Oncogene. 2010, vol 29, pp 285-296.

[300]  Setiawati H, et al. "Effect of Chilli Pepper (Capsicum frutescens L.) on the Bleeding Time, Coagulation Time, and Platelet's Amount of Rats." Publikasi Ilmiah. 2012-06
Also appeared in: INTERNATIONAL CONFERENCE RESEARCH AND APPLICATION ON TRADITIONAL, COMPLEMENTARY, AND ALTERNATIVE MEDICINE IN HEALTH CARE.

[301]  Mason L, et al. "Systematic review of topical capsaicin for the treatment of chronic pain." BMJ. 2004, vol 328, p 991.

[302]  Romero-Matos G. "Devastating treatment against HIV/AIDS with Capsaicin." US Patent. US2004/0224037 A1. Date: Nov 11, 2004.

[303]  Lee SS and Sharkey KA. "Capsaicin treatment blocks development of hyperkinetic circulation in portal hypertensive and cirrhotic rats." AJP. 1993, vol 264(5), pp G868-G873.

[304]  Marks DR, et al. "A double-blind placebo-controlled trial of intranasal capsaicin for cluster headache." Cephalalgia. 1993, vol 13(2), pp 114-116.

[305]  Kyung Min yang, et al. "Capsaicin induces apoptosis by generating reactive oxygen species and disrupting mitochondrial transmembrane potential in human colon cancer cell lines." Cellular & Molecular Biology Letters. 2009, vol 14(3), pp 497-510.

[306]  Tandan R, et al. "Topical Capsaicin in Painful Diabetic Neuropathy: Controlled Study With Long-Term Follow-Up." <u>Diabetes Care.</u> 1992, vol 15, pp 8-14.

[307]  De Silva V, et al. "Evidence for the efficacy of complementary and alternative medicines in the management of fibromyalgia: a systematic review." <u>Rheumatology.</u> 2010, vol 49(6), pp 1063-1068.

[308]  MN Satyanarayana. "Capsaicin and Gastric Ulcers." <u>Critical Reviews in Food Science and Nutrition.</u> 2006, vol 46(4), pp 275-328.

[309]  Simpson DM, et al. "Controlled trial of high-concentration capsaicin patch for treatment of painful HIV neuropathy." <u>Neurology.</u> 2008, vol 70(24), pp 2305-2313.

[310]  Romero-Matos G. "Devastating treatment against HIV/AIDS with Capsaicin." <u>US Patent.</u> US2004/0224037 A1. Date: Nov 11, 2004.

[311]  Ibid.

[312]  Sampathkumar P, et al. "Herpes Zoster (Shingles) and Postherpetic Neuralgia." <u>Mayo Clin Proc.</u> 2009, vol 84(3), pp 274-280.

[313]  Lee SS and Sharkey KA. "Capsaicin treatment blocks development of hyperkinetic circulation in portal hypertensive and cirrhotic rats." <u>AJP.</u> 1993, vol 264(5), pp G868-G873.

[314]  Brown KC, et al. "Capsaicin Displays Anti-Proliferative Activity against Human Small Cell Lung Cancer in Cell Culture and Nude Mice Models via the E2F Pathway." <u>PLOS Science.</u> 2010

[315]  Franco-Cereceda A and Liska J. "Potential of Calcitonin Gene-Related Peptide in Coronary Heart Disease." <u>Pharmacology.</u> 2000, vol 60(1), pp 108.

[316]  Ip SW, et al. "Capsaicin mediates apoptosis in human nasopharyngeal carcinoma NPC-TW 039 cells through mitochondrial depolarization and endoplasmic reticulum stress." <u>Hum Exp Toxicol.</u> 2011, vol 31(6),  pp 539-549.

[317]  N Jancso, et al. "Direct Evidence for Neurogenic Inflammation and its Prevention by Denervation and by Pretreatment with Capsaicin." <u>Br J Pharmac Chemother.</u> 1967, vol 31, pp138-151.

[318]   Szallasi A. "Vanilloid (Capsaicin) Receptors in Health and Disease." <u>AJCP.</u> 2002, vol 118, pp 110-121.

[319]   Rains C and Bryson HM. "Topical Capsaicin." <u>Drugs & Aging.</u> 1995, vol 7(4), pp 317-328.

[320]   Zhang, R. et al. "In vitro and in vivo induction of apoptosis by capsaicin in pancreatic cancer cells is mediated through ROS generation and mitochondrial death pathway." <u>Apoptosis.</u> 2008, vol 13 (12), pp 1465-1478

[321]   "Which Treatment for Postherpetic Neuralgia?" (PLoS Med 2(7): e238. Doi:10.1371/journal.pmed.0020238) <u>Plos Science.</u>

[322]   Mori A. et al. "Capsaicin, a Component of Red Peppers, Inhibit's the Growth of Androgen-Independent, p53 Mutant Prostate Cancer Cells." <u>The Journal of Cancer Research</u>. 2006. Vol 66; p 3222

[323]   Kober A, et al. "Local Active Warming: An Effective Treatment for Pain, Anxiety and Nausea Caused by Renal Colic." <u>Journal of Urology.</u> 2003, vol 170(3), pp 741-744.

[324]   Ibid.

[325]   Ibid.

[326]   Carson-DeWitt R. "Medications for Shingles." <u>EBSCO Publishing</u>. 2007. http://www.empowher.com/media/reference/medications-shingles

[327]   Stammberger H and Wolf G. "Headaches and sinus disease: the endoscopic approach." <u>Ann Otol Rhinol Laryngol Suppl.</u> 1988, vol 134, pp 3-23.

[328]   Macfarlane R, et al. "Chronic Trigeminal Ganglionectomy or Topical Capsaicin Application to Pial Vessels Attenuates Postocclusive Cortical Hyperemia but Does Not Influence Postischemic Hypoperfusion." <u>Journal of Celebral Blook Fow & Metabolism.</u> 1991, vol 11, pp 261-271.

[329]   Ellison N, et al. "Phase III placebo-controlled trial of capsaicin cream in the management of surgical neuropathic pain in cancer patients." <u>JCO.</u> 1997, vol 15(8), pp 2974-2980.

[330]  Szallasi A. "Vanilloid (Capsaicin) Receptors in Health and Disease." <u>AJCP.</u> 2002, vol 118, pp 110-121.

[331]  Stammberger H and Wolf G. "Headaches and sinus disease: the endoscopic approach." <u>Ann Otol Rhinol Laryngol Suppl.</u> 1988, vol 134, pp 3-23.

[332]  Jih-Pyang Wang et al. "Antithemostatic and antthrombotic effects of capsaicin in comparison with aspirin and indomethacin." <u>Thrombosis Research.</u> 1985, vol 37 (6) pp 669-679

[333]  Caterina MJ, et al. "The capsaicin receptor: a heat-activated ion channel in the pain pathway." <u>Nature.</u> 1997, vol 389, pp 816-824.

[334]  Ghilardi JR, et al. "Selective Blockade of the Capsaicin Receptor TRPV1 Attenuates Bone Cancer Pain." <u>Journal of Neuroscience.</u> 2005, vol 25(12), pp 3126-3131.

[335]  Mori A. et al. "Capsaicin, a Component of Red Peppers, Inhibit's the Growth of Androgen-Independent, p53 Mutant Prostate Cancer Cells." <u>The Journal of Cancer Research</u>. 2006. Vol 66; p 3222

[336]  Pegorini S, et al. "Capsaicin exhibits neuroprotective effects in a model of transient global cerebral ischemia in Mongolian gerbils." <u>BJP.</u> 2005, vol 144(5), pp 727-735.

[337]  Oxford University. "More than Spice: Capsaicin in Hot Chili Peppers Makes Tumor Cells Commit Suicide." <u>JNCI J Natl Cancer Inst</u>. Vol 94 (17), pp 1263-1265

[338]  Jih-Pyang Wang et al. Antithemostatic and antthrombotic effects of capsaicin in comparison with aspirin and indomethacin. <u>Thrombosis Research.</u> 1985, vol 37 (6) pp 669-679

[339]  Setiawati H, et al. "Effect of Chilli Pepper (Capsicum frutescens L.) on the Bleeding Time, Coagulation Time, and Platelet's Amount of Rats." <u>Publikasi Ilmiah</u>. 2012-06
Also appeared in: INTERNATIONAL CONFERENCE RESEARCH AND APPLICATION ON TRADITIONAL, COMPLEMENTARY, AND ALTERNATIVE MEDICINE IN HEALTH CARE.

340  Sampathkumar P, et al. "Herpes Zoster (Shingles) and Postherpetic Neuralgia." <u>Mayo Clin Proc.</u> 2009, vol 84(3), pp 274-280.

341  Keith M. Henry. Cayenne Pepper - Stop a heart attack fast. Nov 30, 2010. http://www.naturalnews.com/030566_cayenne_pepper_heart_attack.html

342  Lim GP, et al. "The Curry Spice Curcumin Reduces Oxidative Damage and Amyloid Pathology in an Alzheimer Transgenic Mouse." <u>The Journal of Neuroscience.</u> 2001, vol 21(21), pp 8370-8377.

343  Pullakhandam R, et al. "Binding and stabilization of transthyretin by curcumin." <u>Archives of Biochemistry and Biophysics.</u> 2009, vol 485(2), pp 115-119.

344  Lal B, et al. "Efficacy of Curcumin in the Management of Chronic Anterior Uveitis." <u>Phytotherapy Research.</u> 1999, vol 13(4), pp 318-322.

345  Goel A, et al. "Curcumin as *"Curecumin"*: From kitchen to clinic." <u>Biochemical Pharmacology.</u> 2008, vol 75(4), pp 787-809.

346  Ibid.

347  Wongcharoen W and Phrommintikul A. "The protective role of curcumin in cardiovascular diseases." <u>International Journal of Cardiology.</u> 2009, vol 133(3), pp 145-151.

348  Strofer M, et al. "Curcumin Decreases Survival of Hep3B Liver and MCF-7 Breast Cancer Cells." <u>Strahlentherapie und Onkologie.</u> 2011, vol 187(7), pp 393-400.

349  Wongcharoen W and Phrommintikul A. "The protective role of curcumin in cardiovascular diseases." <u>International Journal of Cardiology.</u> 2009, vol 133(3), pp 145-151.

350  Goel A, et al. "Curcumin as *"Curecumin"*: From kitchen to clinic." <u>Biochemical Pharmacology.</u> 2008, vol 75(4), pp 787-809.

351  Bengmark S, et al. "Plant-derived health - the effects of turmeric and curcuminoids." <u>Nutr Hosp.</u> 2009, vol 24(3).

352  Ibid.

[353]   Ibid.

[354]   Johnson JJ and Muktar H. "Curcumin for chemoprevention of colon cancer." <u>Cancer Letters.</u> 2007, vol 255(2), pp 170-181.

[355]   Bengmark S, et al. "Plant-derived health - the effects of turmeric and curcuminoids." <u>Nutr Hosp.</u> 2009, vol 24(3).

[356]   Wongcharoen W and Phrommintikul A. "The protective role of curcumin in cardiovascular diseases." <u>International Journal of Cardiology.</u> 2009, vol 133(3), pp 145-151.

[357]   Goel A, et al. "Curcumin as "Curecumin": From kitchen to clinic." <u>Biochemical Pharmacology.</u> 2008, vol 75(4), pp 787-809.

[358]   Wongcharoen W and Phrommintikul A. "The protective role of curcumin in cardiovascular diseases." <u>International Journal of Cardiology.</u> 2009, vol 133(3), pp 145-151.

[359]   Goel A, et al. "Curcumin as "Curecumin": From kitchen to clinic." <u>Biochemical Pharmacology.</u> 2008, vol 75(4), pp 787-809.

[360]   Ibid.

[361]   Bengmark S, et al. "Plant-derived health - the effects of turmeric and curcuminoids." <u>Nutr Hosp.</u> 2009, vol 24(3).

[362]   Strofer M, et al. "Curcumin Decreases Survival of Hep3B Liver and MCF-7 Breast Cancer Cells." <u>Strahlentherapie und Onkologie.</u> 2011, vol 187(7), pp 393-400.

[363]   Pillai GR, et al. "Induction of apoptosis in human lung cancer cells by curcumin." <u>Cancer Letters.</u> 2004, vol 208(2), pp 163-170.

[364]   Shishodia S, et al. "Curcumin (diferuloylmethane) inhibits constitutive NF-κB activation, induces G1/S arrest, suppresses proliferation, and induces apoptosis in mantle cell lymphoma ." <u>Biochemical Pharmacology.</u> 2005, vol 70(5), pp 700-713.

[365]   Goel A, et al. "Curcumin as *"Curecumin"*: From kitchen to clinic." <u>Biochemical Pharmacology.</u> 2008, vol 75(4), pp 787-809.

[366]   Ibid.

[367]   Ibid.

[368]   Ibid.

[369]   Ibid.

[370]   Ibid.

[371]   Park C, et al. "Curcumin induces apoptosis and inhibits prostaglandin E(2) production in synovial fibroblasts of patients with rheumatoid arthritis." <u>International Journal of Molecular Medicine.</u> 2007, vol 20(3), pp 365-372.

[372]   Goel A, et al. "Curcumin as *"Curecumin"*: From kitchen to clinic." <u>Biochemical Pharmacology.</u> 2008, vol 75(4), pp 787-809.

[373]   Wongcharoen W and Phrommintikul A. "The protective role of curcumin in cardiovascular diseases." <u>International Journal of Cardiology.</u> 2009, vol 133(3), pp 145-151.

[374]   Goel A, et al. "Curcumin as *"Curecumin"*: From kitchen to clinic." <u>Biochemical Pharmacology.</u> 2008, vol 75(4), pp 787-809.

[375]   Wongcharoen W and Phrommintikul A. "The protective role of curcumin in cardiovascular diseases." <u>International Journal of Cardiology.</u> 2009, vol 133(3), pp 145-151.

[376]   Ibid.

[377]   Goel A, et al. "Curcumin as *"Curecumin"*: From kitchen to clinic." <u>Biochemical Pharmacology.</u> 2008, vol 75(4), pp 787-809.

[378]   Damodaran Chendil, et al. "Curcumin confers radiosensitizing effect in prostate cancer cell line PC-3." <u>Oncogene.</u> 2004, vol 23, pp 1599-1607.

[379]   Goel A, et al. "Curcumin as *"Curecumin"*: From kitchen to clinic." <u>Biochemical Pharmacology.</u> 2008, vol 75(4), pp 787-809.

[380]   Menon LG, et al. "Inhibition of lung metastasis in mice induced by B16F10 melanoma cells by polyphenolic compounds." <u>Cancer Letters.</u> 1995, vol 95(1-2), pp 221-225.

[381]   Rogerio AP, et al. "Anti-inflammatory effects of *Lafoensia pacari* and ellagic acid in a murine model of asthma." <u>European Journal of Pharmacology.</u> 2008, vol 580(1-2), pp 262-270.

[382]   Te-Mao Li, et al. "Ellagic Acid Induced p53/p21 Expression, G1 Arrest and Apoptosis in Human Bladder Cancer T24 Cells." <u>Anticancer Research.</u> 2005, vol 25(2A), pp 971-979.

[383]   Losso JN, et al. "In vitro anti-proliferative activities of ellagic acid." <u>The Journal of Nutritional Biochemistry.</u> 2004, vol 15(11), pp 672-678.

[384]   DA Vattem and K Shetty. "BIOLOGICAL FUNCTIONALITY OF ELLAGIC ACID: A REVIEW." <u>Journal of Food Biochemistry.</u> 2005 (3), pp 234-266.

[385]   DA Vattem and K Shetty. BIOLOGICAL FUNCTIONALITY OF ELLAGIC ACID: A REVIEW. Journal of Food Biochemistry. 2005 (3), pp 234-266.

[386]   Larrosa M, et al. "The dietary hydrolysable tannin punicalagin releases ellagic acid that induces apoptosis in human colon adenocarcinoma Caco-2 cells by using the mitochondrial pathway." <u>The Journal of Nutritional Biochemistry.</u> 2006, vol 17(9), pp 611-625.

[387]   Whitley AC, et al. "Intestinal epithelial cell accumulation of the cancer preventive polyphenol ellagic acid — extensive binding to protein and DNA." <u>Biochemical Pharmacology.</u> 2003, vol 66(6), pp 907-915.

[388]   Johnson JR, et al. "Effect of Maternal Raspberry Leaf Consumption in Rats on Pregnancy Outcome and the Fertility of the Female Offspring." <u>Reproductive Sciences.</u> 2009, vol 16(6), pp 605-609.

[389]   Johnson JR, et al. "Effect of Maternal Raspberry Leaf Consumption in Rats on Pregnancy Outcome and the Fertility of the Female Offspring." <u>Reproductive Sciences.</u> 2009, vol 16(6), pp 605-609.

[390]  Papoutsi Z, et al. "Evaluation of Estrogenic/Antiestrogenic Activity of Ellagic Acid via the Estrogen Receptor Subtypes ERα and Erβ." J Agric Food Chem. 2005, vol 53(20), pp 7715-7720.

[391]  Susanne U Mertens-Talcott and Susan S Percival. Ellagic acid and quercetin interact synergistically with resveratrol in the induction of apoptosis and cause transient cell cycle arrest in human leukemia cells. Cancer Letters. 2005, vol 218 (2), pp 141-151.

[392]  Boukharta M, et al. "Biodistribution of ellagic acid and dose-related inhibition of lung tumorigenesis in A/J mice." 1992, vol 18(2), pp 181-189.

[393]  Turk G, et al. "Improvement of cisplatin-induced injuries to sperm quality, the oxidant-antioxidant system, and the histologic structure of the rat testis by ellagic acid.." Fertility and Sterility.  2008, vol89(5), pp 1474-1481.

[394]  Papoutsi Z, et al. "Evaluation of Estrogenic/Antiestrogenic Activity of Ellagic Acid via the Estrogen Receptor Subtypes ERα and Erβ." J Agric Food Chem. 2005, vol 53(20), pp 7715-7720.

[395]  Carolyn Bell and Susan Hawthorne. "Ellagic acid, pomegranate and prostate cancer — a mini review." Journal of Pharmacy and Pharmacology.  2008, vol 69(2), pp 139-144.

[396]  Akagi K, et al. "Modulating effects of ellagic acid, vanillin and quercetin in a rat medium term multi-organ carcinogenesis model." Cancer Letters.  1995, vol 94(1), pp 113-121.

[397]  Turk G, et al. "Improvement of cisplatin-induced injuries to sperm quality, the oxidant-antioxidant system, and the histologic structure of the rat testis by ellagic acid.." Fertility and Sterility.  2008, vol89(5), pp 1474-1481.

[398]  Ji-Young Bae, et al. "Dietary compound ellagic acid alleviates skin wrinkle and inflammation induced by UV-B irradiation." Experimental Dermatology. 2010, vol 19(8),  pp 3182-e190.

[399]  Rogerio AP, et al. "Anti-inflammatory effects of *Lafoensia pacari* and ellagic acid in a murine model of asthma." European Journal of Pharmacology. 2008, vol 580(1-2), pp 262-270.

400   Boukharta M, et al. "Biodistribution of ellagic acid and dose-related inhibition of lung tumorigenesis in A/J mice." <u>1992, vol 18(2),</u> pp 181-189.

401   Johnson JR, et al. "Effect of Maternal Raspberry Leaf Consumption in Rats on Pregnancy Outcome and the Fertility of the Female Offspring." <u>Reproductive Sciences.</u>  2009, vol 16(6), pp 605-609.

402   Kang MK, et al. "Gallic acid induces neuronal cell death through activation of c-Jun N-terminal kinase and downregulation of Bcl-2." <u>Ann N Y Acad Sci.</u> 2009, vol 1171, pp 514-520.

403   Jang A, et al. "Comparison of hypolipidemic activity of synthetic gallic acid–linoleic acid ester with mixture of gallic acid and linoleic acid, gallic acid, and linoleic acid on high-fat diet induced obesity in C57BL/6 Cr Slc mice." <u>Chemico-</u>

404   Harput US, et al. Cytotoxic and antioxidative activities of Plantago lagopus L. and characterization of its bioactive compounds. Food Chem Toxicol. 2012, vol 50 (5), pp 1554-1559.

405   Abdelwahed A, et al. "Study of antimutagenic and antioxidant activities of Gallic acid and 1,2,3,4,6-pentagalloylglucose from *Pistacia lentiscus*: Confirmation by microarray expression profiling." <u>Chemico-Biological Interations.</u> 2007, vol 165(1), pp 1-13.

406   Seeram NP, et al. "In vitro antiproliferative, apoptotic and antioxidant activities of punicalagin, ellagic acid and a total pomegranate tannin extract are enhanced in combination with other polyphenols as found in pomegranate juice." <u>Journal of Nutritional Biochemistry.</u> 2005, vol 16, pp 360-367.

407  Zhang J, et al. Anti-cancer, anti-diabetic and other pharmacologic and biological activities of penta-galloyl-glucose. Pharm Res. 2009, vol 26 (9), p 2066.

408   Chandramohan RT, et al. Anti-leukemic effects of gallic acid on human leukemia K562 cells: downregulation of COX-2, inhibition of BCR/ABL kinase and NF-?B inactivation. Toxicol In Vitro. 2012, vol 26 (3), pp 396-405.

Yeh RD, et al. Gallic acid induces G0/G1 phase arrest and apoptosis in human leukemia HL-60 cells through inhibiting cyclin D and E, and activating mitochondria-dependent pathway. Anticancer Res. 2011, vol 31 (9), pp 2821-2832.

[409]  Kyung-Ghul Choi, et al. "Gallic Acid Suppresses Lipopolysaccharide-Induced Nuclear Factor-κB Signaling by Preventing RelA Acetylation in A549 Lung Cancer Cells." <u>Molecular Cancer Res.</u> 2009, vol 7, doi:10.1158/1541-7786.MCR-09-0239.

[410]  Nabasree Dasgupta and Bratati De. "Antioxidant activity of *Piper betle* L. leaf extract in vitro." <u>Food Chemistry.</u> 2004, vol 88(2), pp 219-224.

[411]  Russell LH Jr., et al. "Differential cytotoxicity of triphala and its phenolic constituent gallic acid on human prostate cancer LNCap and normal cells." <u>Anticancer Res</u>. 2011, vol 31 (11), pp 3739-3745.

[412]  Jang A, et al. "Comparison of hypolipidemic activity of synthetic gallic acid–linoleic acid ester with mixture of gallic acid and linoleic acid, gallic acid, and linoleic acid on high-fat diet induced obesity in C57BL/6 Cr Slc mice." <u>Chemico-Biological Interactions.</u> 2008, vol 174(2), pp 109-117.

[413]  Zhang J, et al. Anti-cancer, anti-diabetic and other pharmacologic and biological activities of penta-galloyl-glucose. <u>Pharm Res</u>. 2009, vol 26 (9), p 2066.

[414]  Ibid.

[415]  Chandramohan RT, et al. "Anti-leukemic effects of gallic acid on human leukemia K562 cells: downregulation of COX-2, inhibition of BCR/ABL kinase and NF-?B inactivation." <u>Toxicol In Vitro</u>. 2012, vol 26 (3), pp 396-405.

[416]  Abdelwahed A, et al. "Study of antimutagenic and antioxidant activities of Gallic acid and 1,2,3,4,6-pentagalloylglucose from *Pistacia lentiscus*: Confirmation by microarray expression profiling." <u>Chemico-Biological Interations.</u> 2007, vol 165(1), pp 1-13.

[417]  Harput US, et al. "Cytotoxic and antioxidative activities of Plantago lagopus L. and characterization of its bioactive compounds." <u>Food Chem Toxicol</u>. 2012, vol 50 (5), pp 1554-1559.

[418]  Jang A, et al. "Comparison of hypolipidemic activity of synthetic gallic acid–linoleic acid ester with mixture of gallic acid and linoleic acid, gallic acid, and linoleic acid on high-fat diet induced obesity in C57BL/6 Cr Slc mice." <u>Chemico-Biological Interactions.</u> 2008, vol 174(2), pp 109-117.

419   Yuegang Zuo, et al. "Simultaneous determination of catechins, caffeine and gallic acids in green, Oolong, black and pu-erh teas using HPLC with a photodiode array detector." <u>Talanta.</u> 2002, vol 57(2), pp 307-316.

420   Nabasree Dasgupta and Bratati De. "Antioxidant activity of *Piper betle* L. leaf extract in vitro." <u>Food Chemistry.</u> 2004, vol 88(2), pp 219-224.

421   Chiueh CC, et al. "Intracranial microdialysis of salicylic acid to detect hydroxyl radical generation through dopamine autooxidation in the caudate nucleus: Effects of MPP." <u>Free Radical Biology and Medicine.</u> 1992, vol 13(5), pp 581-583.

422   Bhattacharyya M, et al. "Acetyl salicylic acid (aspirin) improves synthesis of maspin and lowers incidence of metastasis in breast cancer patients [corrected]." <u>Cancer Sci</u>. 2010, vol 101 (10), pp 2105-2109.

423   Gasparyan AY, et al. "The Role of Aspirin in Cardiovascular Prevention Implications of Aspirin Resistance." <u>J Am Coll Cardiol.</u> 2008, vol 51(19), pp 1829-1843.

424   McKee SA, et al. "Aspirin Resistance in Cardiovascular Disease: A Review of Prevalence, Mechanisms, and Clinical Significance." <u>Thrombosis and Haemostasis</u>. 2002, vol 88(5), pp 711-715.

425   Thun MJ, et al. "Aspirin use and Reduced Risk of fatal Colon Cancer." <u>The New England Journal of Medicine.</u> 1991, vol 325 (23), pp 1593-1596.

426   JR Paterson and JR Lawrence. "Salicylic acid: a link between aspirin, diet and the prevention of colorectal cancer." <u>QJM.</u> 2001, vol 94(8), pp 445-448.

427   Gasparyan AY, et al. "The Role of Aspirin in Cardiovascular Prevention Implications of Aspirin Resistance." <u>J Am Coll Cardiol.</u> 2008, vol 51(19), pp 1829-1843.

428   Ibid.

429   Rodriguez-Cerdeira C and Sanchez-Blanco E. "Glycolic acid 15% plus salicylic acid 2%: a new therapeutic pearl for facial flat warts." <u>J Clin Aesthet Dermatol</u>. 2011, vol 4(9), pp 62-64.

[430]  Gasparyan AY, et al. "The Role of Aspirin in Cardiovascular Prevention Implications of Aspirin Resistance." <u>J Am Coll Cardiol.</u> 2008, vol 51(19), pp 1829-1843.

[431]  Ibid.

[432]  Paqe BD, et al. "Small molecule STAT5-SH2 domain inhibitors exhibit potent antileukemia activity. " <u>J Med Chem</u>. 2012, vol 55(3), pp 1047-1055.

[433]  Chiueh CC, et al. "Intracranial microdialysis of salicylic acid to detect hydroxyl radical generation through dopamine autooxidation in the caudate nucleus: Effects of MPP." <u>Free Radical Biology and Medicine.</u> 1992, vol 13(5), pp 581-583.

[434]  Gianocotti A, et al.  Efficacy of three different antithrombotic regimens on pregnancy outcome in pregnant women affected by recurrent pregnancy loss. J Matern Fetal Neonatal Med. 2012, vol 25(7), pp 1191-1194.

[435]  Gasparyan AY, et al. "The Role of Aspirin in Cardiovascular Prevention Implications of Aspirin Resistance." <u>J Am Coll Cardiol.</u> 2008, vol 51(19), pp 1829-1843.

[436]  Zhang T, et al. A novel naturally occurring salicylic acid analogue acts as an anti-inflammatory agent by inhibiting nuclear factor-kappaB activity in RAW264.7 macrophages. Mol Pharm. 2012, vol 9 (3), pp 671-677.

[437]  Shabir G, et al. Antioxidant and antimicrobial attributes and phenolics of different solvent extracts from leaves, flowers and bark of Gold Mohar [Delonix regia (Bojer ex Hook.) Raf]. Molecules. 2011, vol 16(9), pp 7302-7319.

[438]  Shabir G, et al. Antioxidant and antimicrobial attributes and phenolics of different solvent extracts from leaves, flowers and bark of Gold Mohar [Delonix regia (Bojer ex Hook.) Raf]. Molecules. 2011, vol 16(9), pp 7302-7319.

[439]  Gasparyan AY, et al. "The Role of Aspirin in Cardiovascular Prevention Implications of Aspirin Resistance." <u>J Am Coll Cardiol.</u> 2008, vol 51(19), pp 1829-1843.

[440]  Nulton-Persson AC, et al. "Inhibition of Cardiac Mitochondrial Respiration by Salicylic Acid and Acetylsalicylate." <u>Journal of Cardiovascular Pharmacology.</u> 2004, vol 44(5), pp 591-595.

[441]  Calixto JB, et al. "Pharmacological Actions of Tannic Acid. I. Effects on Isolated Smooth and Cardiac Muscles and on Blood Pressure." Planta Med. 1986, vol 52(1), pp 32-35.

[442]  Blalock A. "EXPERIMENTAL SHOCK: VII. THE IMPORTANCE OF THE LOCAL LOSS OF FLUID IN THE PRODUCTION OF THE LOW BLOOD PRESSURE AFTER BURNS." Arch Surg. 1931, vol 22, pp 610-616.

[443]  Beck CS and Powers JH. "Burns Treated by Tannic Acid." Ann Surg. vol 84(1), pp 19-36.

[444]  El-Ghitany EM and Abd El Salam MM. Environmental intervention for house dust mite control in childhood bronchial asthma. Environ Health Prev Med. 2012, vol 17(5), pp 377-384.

[445]  Sanchez-Tena S, et al. Hamamelitannin from witch hazel (Hamamelis virginiana) displays specific cytotoxic activity against colon cancer cells. J Nt Pro. 2012, vol 75(1), pp 26-33.

[446]  El-Ghitany EM and Abd El Salam MM. Environmental intervention for house dust mite control in childhood bronchial asthma. Environ Health Prev Med. 2012, vol 17(5), pp 377-384.

[447]  Krisper P, et al. "The use of Tannin from Chestnut (Castanea Vesca)." Plant Polyphenols  Basic Life Sciences. 1992, vol 59, pp 1013-1019.

[448]  Krisper P, et al. "The use of Tannin from Chestnut (Castanea Vesca)." Plant Polyphenols  Basic Life Sciences. 1992, vol 59, pp 1013-1019.

[449]  Fahim MS. "TOPICAL APPLICATION OF MEDICATION BY ULTRASOUND WITH COUPLING AGENT." US Patent. 933,205  Date: Aug. 14, 1998.

[450]  Ibid.

[451]  Otari KV, et al. Protective effect of aqueous extract of Spinacia oleracea leaves in experimental paradigms of inflammatory bowel disease. Inflammopharmacology. 2012, vol 20(5), pp 277-287.

452   Miyamoto H, et al. ALTA injection sclerosing therapy:non-excisional treatment of internal hemorrhoids.
Hepatogastroenterology. 2012, vol 59(113), pp 77-80.


453   Krisper P, et al. "The use of Tannin from Chestnut (Castanea Vesca)." Plant Polyphenols  Basic Life Sciences. 1992, vol 59, pp 1013-1019.


454   Fahim MS. "TOPICAL APPLICATION OF MEDICATION BY ULTRASOUND WITH COUPLING AGENT." US Patent. 933,205  Date: Aug. 14, 1998.


455   Smith DB and Jacobson BH. "Effect of a blend of comfrey root extract (*Symphytum officinale* L.) and tannic acid creams in the treatment of osteoarthritis of the knee: randomized, placebo-controlled, double-blind, multiclinical trials." Journal of Chiropractic Medicine. 2011, vol 10(3), pp 147-156.


456   Khanna S, et al. "DERMAL WOUND HEALING PROPERTIES OF REDOX-ACTIVE GRAPE SEED PROANTHOCYANIDINS." Free Radical Biology & Medicine. 2002, vol 33(8), pp 1089-1096.


457   Kim JM, et al. Heterologous expression of a tannic acid-inducible laccase3 of Cryphonectria parasitica in Saccharomyces cerevisiae. BMC Biotechnol. 2010, vol 10, p 18.


458   Shen M, et al. Targeting tumor ubiquitin-proteasome pathway with polyphenols for chemosensitization. Anticancer Agents Med Chem. 2012, vol 12(8), pp 891-901.


459   Zhang XF, et al. Tannic acid inhibited norovirus binding to HBGA receptors, a study of 50 Chinese medicinal herbs. Bioorg Med Chem. 2012, vol 20(4), pp 1616-1623.


460   Beck CS and Powers JH. "Burns Treated by Tannic Acid." Ann Surg. vol 84(1), pp 19-36.


461   Krisper P, et al. "The use of Tannin from Chestnut (Castanea Vesca)." Plant Polyphenols  Basic Life Sciences. 1992, vol 59, pp 1013-1019.


462   Nam Deuk Kim, et al. Chemopreventive and adjuvant therapeutic potential of pomegranate (Punica granatum) for human breast cancer. Breast Cancer Research and Treatment. 2002, vol 71 (3), pp 203-217.

[463]  Li H, et al. Review in the studies on tannins activity of cancer prevention and anticancer. Ahong Yao Cai. 2003, vol 26 (6), pp 444-448.

[464]  Keiji Funatogawa, et al. Antibacterial Activity of Hydrolyzable Tannins derived from Medicinal Plants against Helicobacter pylori. Microbio Immunol. 2004, vol 48 (4), pp 251-261.

[465]  Harnett SM et al. "Anti-HIV activities of organic and aqueous extracts of *Sutherlandia frutescens* and *Lobostemon trigonus*." Journal of Ethnopharmacology. 2005, vol 96(1-2), pp 113-119.

[466]  Keiji Funatogawa, et al. Antibacterial Activity of Hydrolyzable Tannins derived from Medicinal Plants against Helicobacter pylori. Microbio Immunol. 2004, vol 48 (4), pp 251-261.

[467]  Zongchun Yi, et al. Inhibitory effect of tellimagrandin I on chemically induced differentiation of human leukemia K562 cells. Toxicology Letters. 2004, vol 147 (2), pp 109-119.

[468]  Pantuck AJ, et al. Phase II Study of Pomegranate Juice for Men with Rising Prostate-Specific Antigen following Surgery or Radiation for Prostate Cancer. Clin Cancer Res. 2006, vol 12 p 4018.

[469]  Meenakshi Shukla, et al. Consumption of Hydrolyzable Tannins Rich Pomegranate Extract (POMx) Suppresses Inflammation and Joint Damage In Rheumatoid Arthritis. Nutrition. 2008, vol 24 (7-8), pp 733-743.

[470]  Hisanori Akiyama, et al. Antibacterial action of several tannins against *Staphylococcus aureus*. J Antimicrob Chemother. 2001, vol 48 (4), pp 487-491.

[471]  Gali-Muhtasib HU, et al. "Tannins Protect Against Skin Tumor Promotion Induced by Ultraviolet-B Radiation in Hairless Mice." Nutrition and Cancer. 2000, vol 37(1), pp 73-77.

[472]  Kuroda Y and Inoue T. "Antimutagenesis by factors affecting DNA repair in bacteria." Mutation Research/Fundamental and Molecular Mechanisms of Mutagenesis. 1988, vol 202(2), pp 387-391.

[473]   Sakagami H, et al. Cytotoxic activity of hydrolyzable tannins against human oral tumor cell lines — A possible mechanism. Phytomedicine. 2000, vol 7 (1), pp 39-47.

[474]   Kumar SS, et al. "Inhibition of Peroxynitrite-Mediated Reactions by Vanillin." J Agric Food Chem. 2004, vol 52(1), pp 139-145.

[475]   Seong Jin Yu, et al. "Gastrodia elata Blume and an Active Component, p-Hydroxybenzyl Alcohol Reduce Focal Ischemic Brain Injury through Antioxidant Related Gene Expressions." Biological and Pharmaceutical Bulletin. 2005, vol 28(6), pp 1016-1020.

[476]   Kriengsak Lirdprapamongkol et al.  "Vanillin suppresses in vitro invasion and in vivo metastasis of mouse breast cancer cells." European Journal of Pharmaceutical Sciences. 2005, vol 25(1), pp 57-65.

[477]   Kriengsak Lirdprapamongkol et al. "Vanillin Suppresses Metastatic Potential of Human Cancer Cells through PI3K Inhibition and Decreases Angiogenesis in Vivo." J Agric and Food Chem. 2009, vol 57(8), pp 3055-3063.

[478]   Seong Jin Yu, et al. "Gastrodia elata Blume and an Active Component, p-Hydroxybenzyl Alcohol Reduce Focal Ischemic Brain Injury through Antioxidant Related Gene Expressions." Biological and Pharmaceutical Bulletin. 2005, vol 28(6), pp 1016-1020.

[479]   Deb J, et al. "Activity of aspirin analogues and vanillin in a human colorectal cancer cell line." Oncol Rep. 2011, vol 26(3), pp 557-565.

[480]   Seong Jin Yu, et al. "Gastrodia elata Blume and an Active Component, p-Hydroxybenzyl Alcohol Reduce Focal Ischemic Brain Injury through Antioxidant Related Gene Expressions." Biological and Pharmaceutical Bulletin. 2005, vol 28(6), pp 1016-1020.

[481]   Yemiş, Gökçe Polat, et al. "Effect of Vanillin, Ethyl Vanillin, and Vanillic Acid on the Growth and Heat Resistance of Cronobacter Species." Journal of Food Protection. 2011, vol 74(12), pp 2062-2069.

[482]  Seong Jin Yu, et al. "Gastrodia elata Blume and an Active Component, p-Hydroxybenzyl Alcohol Reduce Focal Ischemic Brain Injury through Antioxidant Related Gene Expressions." <u>Biological and Pharmaceutical Bulletin.</u> 2005, vol 28(6), pp 1016-1020.

[483]  Wagner H, et al. "Rhizoma Gastrodiae Tianma." <u>Chromatographic Fingerprint Analysis of Herbal Medicines.</u> 2011, pp 255-262.

[484]  Ibid.

[485]  Kumar SS, et al. "Inhibition of Peroxynitrite-Mediated Reactions by Vanillin." J Agric Food Chem. 2004, vol 52(1), pp 139-145.

[486]  Vinay Dwivedi, et al. "Comparative Anticancer Potential of Clove (gium aromaticum) - an Indian spice - Against Cancer Cell Lines of Various Anatomical Origin." <u>Asian Pacific J Cancer pre.</u> 1989-1993, vol 12.

[487]  Wagner H, et al. "Rhizoma Gastrodiae Tianma." <u>Chromatographic Fingerprint Analysis of Herbal Medicines.</u> 2011, pp 255-262.

[488]  Abdulmalik O, et al. "Crystallographic analysis of human hemoglobin elucidates the structural basis of the potent and dual antisickling activity of pyridyl derivatives of vanillin." <u>Acta Crystallogr D Biol Crystallogr.</u> 2011, vol 67(Pt11), pp 920-928.

[489]  Wagner H, et al. "Rhizoma Gastrodiae Tianma." <u>Chromatographic Fingerprint Analysis of Herbal Medicines.</u> 2011, pp 255-262.

[490]  Ibid.

[491]  Kuroda Y and Inoue T. "Antimutagenesis by factors affecting DNA repair in bacteria." <u>Mutation Research/Fundamental and Molecular Mechanisms of Mutagenesis.</u> 1988, vol 202(2), pp 387-391.

[492]  Wagner H, et al. "Rhizoma Gastrodiae Tianma." <u>Chromatographic Fingerprint Analysis of Herbal Medicines.</u> 2011, pp 255-262.

[493]  Ibid.

[494]  Abdulmalik O, et al. "Crystallographic analysis of human hemoglobin elucidates the structural basis of the potent and dual antisickling activity of pyridyl derivatives of vanillin." Acta Crystallogr D Biol Crystallogr. 2011, vol 67(Pt11), pp 920-928.

[495]  Seong Jin Yu, et al. "Gastrodia elata Blume and an Active Component, p-Hydroxybenzyl Alcohol Reduce Focal Ischemic Brain Injury through Antioxidant Related Gene Expressions." Biological and Pharmaceutical Bulletin. 2005, vol 28(6), pp 1016-1020.

[496]  Wagner H, et al. "Rhizoma Gastrodiae Tianma." Chromatographic Fingerprint Analysis of Herbal Medicines. 2011, pp 255-262.

[497]  Seong Jin Yu, et al. "Gastrodia elata Blume and an Active Component, p-Hydroxybenzyl Alcohol Reduce Focal Ischemic Brain Injury through Antioxidant Related Gene Expressions." Biological and Pharmaceutical Bulletin. 2005, vol 28(6), pp 1016-1020.

[498]  Wagner H, et al. "Rhizoma Gastrodiae Tianma." Chromatographic Fingerprint Analysis of Herbal Medicines. 2011, pp 255-262.

[499]  Andrade JP and Assunção M. "Protective effects of chronic green tea consumption on age-related neurodegeneration." Curr Pharm Des. 2012, vol 18(1), pp 4-14.

[500]  Mandel SA et al. "Simultaneous Manipulation of Multiple Brain Targets by Green Tea Catechins: A Potential Neuroprotective Strategy for Alzheimer and Parkinson Diseases." CNS Neuroscience & Therapeutics. 2008, vol 14 (4) pp 352-365.

[501]  Li-Quin Tang, et al. "Effects and mechanisms of catechin for adjuvant arthritis in rats." Advances in Therapy. 2007, vol 24(3), pp 679-690.

[502]  Nurulain T Zaveri. Green tea and its polyphenolic catechins: Medicinal uses in cancer and no cancer  applications. Life Sciences. 2008, vol 78, pp 2073-2080.

[503]  Sartippour MR, et al. Green Tea and its Catechins inhibit Breast Cancer Xenografts. Nutrition and Cancer. 2001, vol 40 (2).

[504]   Nurulain T Zaveri. Green tea and its polyphenolic catechins: Medicinal uses in cancer and no cancer  applications. Life Sciences. 2008, vol 78, pp 2073-2080.

[505]   Mandel SA et al. Simultaneous Manipulation of Multiple Brain Targets by Green Tea Catechins: A Potential Neuroprotective Strategy for Alzheimer and Parkinson Diseases. CNS Neuroscience & Therapeutics. 2008, vol 14 (4) pp 352-365.

[506]   Tomonori Nagao, et al. "A Catechin-rich Beverage Improves Obesity and Blood Glucose Control in Patients With Type 2 Diabetes." 2009 North American Assn for the Study of Obesity. Obesity. 2009, vol 17 (2), pp 310-317.

[507]   Osakabe N, et al. "Ingestion of Proanthocyanidins Derived from Cacao Inhibits Diabetes-Induced Cataract Formation in Rats." Exp Biol Med. 2004, vol 229(1), pp 33-39.

[508]   Nagao T, et al. "A Catechin-rich Beverage Improves Obesity and Blood Glucose Control in Patients With Type 2 Diabetes." Obesity. 2009, vol 17(2), pp 310-317.

[509]   Bolduc V, et al. "Catechin prevents severe dyslipidemia-associated changes in wall biomechanics of cerebral arteries in LDLr-/-:hApoB+/+ mice and improves cerebral blood flow." Am J Physiol Heart Circ Physiol. 2012, vol 302(6), pp H1330-1339.

[510]   Nagao T, et al. "Ingestion of a tea rich in catechins leads to a reduction in body fat and malondialdehyde-modified LDL in men." Am J Clin Nutr. 2005, vol 81(1), pp 122-129.

[511]   Nath, S et al. "Catechins protect neurons against mitochondrial toxins and HIV proteins via activation of the BDNF pathway." Journal of NeuroVirology. 2012, vol 18 (6), pp 444-455.

[512]   Nurulain T Zaveri. Green tea and its polyphenolic catechins: Medicinal uses in cancer and no cancer  applications. Life Sciences. 2008, vol 78, pp 2073-2080.

[513]   Kakuda T. "Neuroprotective effects of the green tea components theanine and catechins." Biol Pharm Bull. 2002, vol 25(12), pp 1513-1528.

514   Arts ICW, et al. "Catechin intake might explain the inverse relation between tea consumption and ischemic heart disease: the Zutphen Elderly Study." <u>Am J Clin Nutr.</u> 2001, vol 74(2), pp 227-232.

515   Holt RR, et al. Chocolate Consumption and Platelet Function. <u>JAMA.</u> 2002, vol 287 (17), pp 2212-2287.

516   Liang G, et al. "Green tea catechins augment the antitumor activity of doxorubicin in an in vivo mouse model for chemoresistant liver cancer." <u>Int J Oncol</u>. 2010, vol 37(1), pp 111-123.
http://www.ncbi.nlm.nih.gov/pubmed/20514403

517   K Imai and K Nakachi. "Cross sectional study of effects of drinking green tea on cardiovascular and liver diseases." <u>BMJ.</u> 1995, vol 310, p 693.

518   Choi JI, et al. "Role of neuronal nitric oxide synthase in the antiallodynic effects of intrathecal EGCG in a neuropathic pain rat model." <u>Neurosci Lett.</u> 2012, vol 510(1), pp 53-57.

519   Nagao T, et al. "Ingestion of a tea rich in catechins leads to a reduction in body fat and malondialdehyde-modified LDL in men." <u>Am J Clin Nutr.</u> 2005, vol 81(1), pp 122-129.

520   Mandel SA et al. Simultaneous Manipulation of Multiple Brain Targets by Green Tea Catechins: A Potential Neuroprotective Strategy for Alzheimer and Parkinson Diseases. CNS Neuroscience & Therapeutics. 2008, vol 14 (4) pp 352-365.

521   Bettuzzi S, et al. Chemoprevention of Human Prostate Cancer by Oral Administration of Green Tea Catechins in Volunteers with High-Grade Prostate Intraepithelial Neoplasia: A Preliminary Report from a One-Year Proof-of-Principle Study. Cancer Res. 2006, vol 66, p 1234.

522   Hibasami H, et al. Induction of apoptosis in human stomach cancer cells by green tea catechins. Oncology Reports. 1998, vol 5 (2), pp 527-529.

523   Foods high in Catechins. Livestrong.
http://www.livestrong.com/article/478075-foods-high-in-catechins/

[524]    Cho SY, Park PJ, Shin HJ, et al,  "(-)-Catechin suppresses expression of Kruppel-like factor 7 and increases expression and secretion of adiponectin protein in 3T3-L1 cells." <u>Am. J. Physiol. Endocrinol. Metab</u>. 2007, vol 292 (4)

     Matsumoto N, et al. "Cloning the cDNA for a new human zinc finger protein defines a group of closely related Krüppel-like transcription factors." <u>The Journal of Biological Chemistry.</u> 1998, vol 273 (43).

[525]    Lee HJ, et al. Anti-influenza virus activity of green tea by-products in vitro and efficacy against influenza virus infection in chickens." <u>Poult Sci.</u> 2012, vol 91(1), pp 66-73.

[526]    Kakuda T. "Neuroprotective effects of the green tea components theanine and catechins." <u>Biol Pharm Bull.</u> 2002, vol 25(12), pp 1513-1528.

[527]    Hirose M, et al. "Green tea catechins enhance tumor development in the colon without effects in the lung or thyroid after pretreatment with 1,2-Dimethylhydrazine or 2,2'-dihydroxy-di-n-propylnitrosamine in male F344 rats." <u>Cancer Letters.</u> 2001, vol 168(1), pp 23-29.

[528]    Donovan JL, et al. "(+)-Catechin is more bioavailable than (-)-catechin: Relevance to the bioavailability of catechin from cocoa." <u>Free Radical Research.</u> 2006, vol 40(10), pp 1029-1034.

[529]    Mandel SA, et al. "Simultaneous Manipulation of Multiple Brain Targets by Green Tea Catechins: A Potential Neuroprotective Strategy for Alzheimer and Parkinson Diseases." <u>CNS Neuroscience & Therapeutics.</u> 2008, vol 14(4), pp 352-365.

[530]    Engler MB and Engler MM. "The Emerging Role of Flavonoid-Rich Cocoa and Chocolate in Cardiovascular Health and Disease." <u>Nutrition Reviews.</u> 2006, vol 64, pp 109-118.

[531]    Thanqapazham RL, et al. "Green tea polyphenols and its constituent epigallocatechin gallate inhibits proliferation of human breast cancer cells in vitro and in vivo." <u>Cancer Lett.</u> 2007, vol 245(1-2), pp 232-241.

[532]    Engler MB and Engler MM. "The Emerging Role of Flavonoid-Rich Cocoa and Chocolate in Cardiovascular Health and Disease." <u>Nutrition Reviews.</u> 2006, vol 64(3), pp 109-118.

533   Ramos S, et al. "Dietary flavanols exert different effects on antioxidant defenses and apoptosis/proliferation in Caco-2 and SW480 colon cancer cells." <u>Toxicol In Vitro</u>. 2011, vol 25(8), pp 1771-1781.

534   Flammer AJ, et al. "Dark Chocolate Improves Coronary Vasomotion and Reduces Platelet Reactivity." <u>Circulation.</u> 2007, vol 116, pp 2376-2382.

535   Rizvi SI and Zaid MA. "Insulin-Like Effect Of (–)Epicatechin On Erythrocyte Membrane Acetylcholinesterase Activity In Type 2 Diabetes Mellitus." <u>Clinical and Experimental Pharmacology and Physiology.</u> 2001, vol 28(9), pp 776-778.

536   Nath S, et al. "Catechins protect neurons against mitochondrial toxins and HIV proteins via activation of the BDNF pathway." <u>Journal of NeuroVirology.</u> 2012, vol 18(6), pp 445-455.
http://link.springer.com/article/10.1007%2Fs13365-012-0122-1

537   Ciesek S, et al. "The green tea polyphenol, epigallocatechin-3-gallate, inhibits hepatitis C virus entry." <u>Hepatology.</u> 2011, vol 54(6), pp 1947-1955.

538   Suganuma M, et al. "Synergistic Effects of (-)-Epigallocatechin Gallate with (-)-Epicatechin, Sulindac, or Tamoxifen on Cancer-preventive Activity in the Human Lung CancerCell Line PC-9." <u>Cancer Res.</u> 1999, vol 59, p 44.

539   Kurbitz C, et al. "Epicatechin gallate and catechin gallate are superior to epigallocatechin gallate in growth suppression and anti-inflammatory activities in pancreatic tumor cells." <u>Cancer Sci</u>. 2011, vol 102(4), pp 728-734.

540   Mandel SA, et al. "Simultaneous Manipulation of Multiple Brain Targets by Green Tea Catechins: A Potential Neuroprotective Strategy for Alzheimer and Parkinson Diseases." <u>CNS Neuroscience & Therapeutics. </u>2008, vol 14(4), pp 352-365.

541   Duhon D, et al. "The polyphenol epigallocatechin-3-gallate affects lipid rafts to block activation of the c-Met receptor in prostate cancer cells." <u>Mol Carcinog.</u> 2010, vol 49(8), pp 739-749.

542   van Praag H, et al. "Plant-Derived Flavanol (-)Epicatechin Enhances Angiogenesis and Retention of Spatial Memory in Mice." <u>Journal of Neuroscience</u>. 2007, vol 27(22), pp 5869-5878.

543   Engler MB and Engler MM. "The Emerging Role of Flavonoid-Rich Cocoa and Chocolate in Cardiovascular Health and Disease." <u>Nutrition Reviews.</u> 2006, vol 64, pp 109-118.
http://onlinelibrary.wiley.com/doi/10.1111/j.1753-4887.2006.tb00194.x/abstract

544   Nath S, et al. "Catechins protect neurons against mitochondrial toxins and HIV proteins via activation of the BDNF pathway." <u>Journal of NeuroVirology.</u> 2012, vol 18(6), pp 445-455.

545   Yu PL, et al. "Effects of catechin, epicatechin and epigallocatechin gallate on testosterone production in rat leydig cells." <u>J Cell Biochem.</u> 2010, vol 110(2), pp 333-342.

546   Engler MB and Engler MM. "The Emerging Role of Flavonoid-Rich Cocoa and Chocolate in Cardiovascular Health and Disease." <u>Nutrition Reviews.</u> 2006, vol 64, pp 109-118.

547   Shah ZA, et al. "The flavanol (-)-epicatechin prevents stroke damage through the Nrf2/HO1 pathway." <u>Journal of Cerebral Blood Flow & Metabolism.</u> 2010, vol 30, pp 1951-1961.

548   Ho Jin Heo and Chang Yong Lee. "Epicatechin and Catechin in Cocoa Inhibit Amyloid β Protein Induced Apoptosis." <u>J Agric Food Chem.</u> 2005, vol 53(6), pp 1445-1448.

549   Kurbitz C, et al. "Epicatechin gallate and catechin gallate are superior to epigallocatechin gallate in growth suppression and anti-inflammatory activities in pancreatic tumor cells." Cancer Sci. 2011, vol 102(4), pp 728-734.

550   Ramos S, et al. "Dietary flavanols exert different effects on antioxidant defenses and apoptosis/proliferation in Caco-2 and SW480 colon cancer cells." <u>Toxicol In Vitro.</u> 2011, vol 25(8), pp 1771-1781.

551   Ho Jin Heo and Chang Yong Lee. "Epicatechin and Catechin in Cocoa Inhibit Amyloid β Protein Induced Apoptosis." <u>J Agric Food Chem.</u> 2005, vol 53(6), pp 1445-1448.

552   Ramos S, et al. "Dietary flavanols exert different effects on antioxidant defenses and apoptosis/proliferation in Caco-2 and SW480 colon cancer cells." Toxicol In Vitro. 2011, vol 25(8), pp 1771-1781.

553   Ho Jin Heo and Chang Yong Lee. "Epicatechin and Catechin in Cocoa Inhibit Amyloid β Protein Induced Apoptosis." J Agric Food Chem. 2005, vol 53(6), pp 1445-1448.

554   Durgo K, et al. "Genotoxic effects of green tea extract on human laryngeal carcinoma cells in vitro." Arh Hig Rada Toksikol. 2011, vol 62(2), pp 139-146.

555   Engler MB and Engler MM. "The Emerging Role of Flavonoid-Rich Cocoa and Chocolate in Cardiovascular Health and Disease." Nutrition Reviews. 2006, vol 64(3), pp 109-118.

556   Weinreb O, et al. "Neurological mechanisms of green tea polyphenols in Alzheimer's and Parkinson's diseases.." The Journal of Nutritional Biochemistry. 2004, vol 15(9), pp 506-516.

557   Keshari RB, et al. "MENTAL HEALTH CHALLENGES AND POSSIBLE SOLUTIONS WITH SPECIAL REFERENCE TO ANXIETY." International Research Journal of Pharmacy. 2011, vol 2(9), pp 1-6.

558   Zhang G, et al. "Anti-cancer activities of tea epigallocatechin-3-gallate in breast cancer patients under radiotherapy." Curr Mol Med. 2012, vol 12(2), pp 163-176.

559   Koo SI and Noh SK. "Green tea as inhibitor of the intestinal absorption of lipids: potential mechanism for its lipid-lowering effect." J Nutr Biochem. 2007, vol 18(3), pp 179-183.

560   Woong Shick Ahn, et al. "A Major Constituent of Green Tea, EGCG, Inhibits the Growth of a Human Cervical Cancer Cell Line, CaSki Cells, through Apoptosis, $G_1$ Arrest, and Regulation of Gene Expression." DNA and Cell Biology. 2003, vol 22(3), pp 217-224.

561   Sachdeva AK, et al. "Protective Effect of Epigallocatechin Gallate in Murine Water-Immersion Stress Model of Chronic Fatigue Syndrome." Basic & Clinical Pharmacology & Toxicology. 2010, vol 106(6), pp 490-496.

[562]   Yanyan Wang, et al. "Green tea epigallocatechin-3-gallate (EGCG) promotes neural progenitor cell proliferation and sonic hedgehog pathway activation during adult hippocampal neurogenesis." <u>Molecular Nutrition & Food Research.</u> 2012, vol 56(8), pp 1292-1303.

[563]   Rizvi SI, et al. "Protective role of tea catechins against oxidation-induced damage of type 2 diabetic erythrocytes." <u>Clin Exp Pharmacol Physiol</u>. 2005, vol 32(1-2), pp 70-75.

[564]   Xu H, et al. "Green tea epigallocatechin-3-gallate inhibits angiogenesis and suppresses vascular endothelial growth factor C/vascular endothelial growth factor receptor 2 expression and signaling in experimental endometriosis in vivo." <u>Fertility and Sterility.</u> 2011, vol 96(4), pp 1021-1028.

[565]   Tao P. "[The inhibitory effects of catechin derivatives on the activities of human immunodeficiency virus reverse transcriptase and DNA polymerases]." <u>Zhongguo Yi Xue Yuan Xue Bao.</u> 1992, vol 14(5), pp 334-338.

[566]   Keshari RB, et al. "MENTAL HEALTH CHALLENGES AND POSSIBLE SOLUTIONS WITH SPECIAL REFERENCE TO ANXIETY." <u>International Research Journal of Pharmacy.</u> 2011, vol 2(9), pp 1-6.

[567]   Weinreb O, et al. "Neurological mechanisms of green tea polyphenols in Alzheimer's and Parkinson's diseases.." <u>The Journal of Nutritional Biochemistry.</u> 2004, vol 15(9), pp 506-516.

[568]   Klaus S, et al. "Epigallocatechin gallate attenuates diet-induced obesity in mice by decreasing energy absorption and increasing fat oxidation." <u>International Journal of Obesity.</u> 2005, vol29, pp 615-623.

[569]   Weinreb O, et al. "Neurological mechanisms of green tea polyphenols in Alzheimer's and Parkinson's diseases.." <u>The Journal of Nutritional Biochemistry.</u> 2004, vol 15(9), pp 506-516.

[570]   Gupta S, et al. "Molecular pathway for (-)-epigallocatechin-3-gallate-induced cell cycle arrest and apoptosis of human prostate carcinoma cells.." <u>Archives of Biochemistry and Biophysics.</u> 2003, vol 410(1), pp 177-185.

[571]  Sakla MS and Lorson CL. "Induction of full-length survival motor neuron by polyphenol botanical compounds." <u>Human Genetics.</u> 2008, vol 122(6), pp 635-643.

[572]  Gillespie K, et al. "Effects of oral consumption of the green tea polyphenol EGCG in a murine model for human Sjogren's syndrome, an autoimmune disease." <u>Life Sciences.</u> 2008, vol 83(17-18), pp 581-588.

[573]  Zhao WH, et al. "Inhibition by epigallocatechin gallate (EGCg) of conjugative R plasmid transfer in Escherichia coli." <u>Journal of Infection and Chemotherapy.</u> 2001, vol 7(3), pp 195-197.

[574]  Xu H, et al. "Green tea epigallocatechin-3-gallate inhibits angiogenesis and suppresses vascular endothelial growth factor C/vascular endothelial growth factor receptor 2 expression and signaling in experimental endometriosis in vivo." <u>Fertility and Sterility.</u> 2011, vol 96(4), pp 1021-1028.

[575]  Kawai Y, et al. "(-)-Epicatechin gallate accumulates in foamy macrophages in human atherosclerotic aorta: implication in the anti-atherosclerotic actions of tea catechins." Biochem Biophys Res Commun. 2008, vol 37(3), pp 527-532.

[576]  Chi Chen, et al. "Epigallocatechin-3-gallate-induced stress signals in HT-29 human colon adenocarcinoma cells." <u>Carcinogenesis.</u> 2003, vol 24(8), pp 1369-1378.

[577]  Engler MB and Engler MM. "The Emerging Role of Flavonoid-Rich Cocoa and Chocolate in Cardiovascular Health and Disease." <u>Nutrition Reviews.</u> 2006, vol 64(3), pp 109-118.

[578]  Hyun Sook Lee, et al. "[6]-Gingerol inhibits metastasis of MDA-MB-231 human breast cancer cells." <u>The Journal of Nutritional Biochemistry.</u> 2008, vol 19(5), pp 313-319.

[579]  Jeong CH, et al. [6]-Gingerol suppresses colon cancer growth by targeting leukotriene A4 hydrolase. Cancer Res. 2009 (13), pp 5584-5591.

[580]  Seong-Ho Lee, et al. "Multiple mechanisms are involved in 6-gingerol-induced cell growth arrest and apoptosis in human colorectal cancer cells." <u>Molecular Carcinogenesis.</u> 2008, vol 47(3), pp 197-208.

581   Ghayur MN, et al. Muscarinic, Ca(++) antagonist and specific butyrylcholinesterase inhibitory activity of dried ginger extract might explain its use in dementia. J Pharm Pharmacol. 2008, vol 60(10), pp 1375-1383.

582   Ishiquro K, et al. Ginger ingredients reduce viability of gastric cancer cells via distinct mechanisms. Biochem Biophys Res Commun. 2007, vol 362(1), pp 218-223.

583   Zeng HL, et al. [Comparative protein analysis of K562 cell apoptosis induced by 6-gingerol]. Zhong Yao Cai. 2010, vol 33(5), p 753-758.

584   Weng CJ, et al. Anti-invasion effects of 6-shogaol and 6-gingerol, two active components in ginger, on human hepatocarcinoma cells. Mol Nutr Food Res. 2010, vol 54(11), pp 1618-1627.

585   Zeng HL, et al. [Comparative protein analysis of K562 cell apoptosis induced by 6-gingerol]. Zhong Yao Cai. 2010, vol 33(5), p 753-758.

586   Rhode J, et al. Ginger inhibits cell growth and modulates angiogenic factors in ovarian cancer cells. BMC Complement Altern Med. 2007, vol 7, p 44.

587   Park YJ, et al. [6]-Gingerol induces cell cycle arrest and cell death of mutant p53-expressing pancreatic cancer cells. Yonsei Med J. 2006, vol 47(5), pp 688-697.

588   Yogeshwer Shukla, et al. "In vitro and in vivo modulation of testosterone mediated alterations in apoptosis related proteins by [6]-gingerol." Molecular Nutrition & Food Research. 2007, vol 51(12), pp 1492-1502.

589   Nonn L, et al. Chemopreventive anti-inflammatory activities of curcumin and other phytochemicals mediated by MAP kinase phosphatase-5 in prostate cells. Carcinogenesis. 2007, vol 28(6), pp 1188-1196.

590   Funk JL, et al. Comparative effects of two gingerol-containing Zingiber officinale extracts on experimental rheumatoid arthritis. J Nat Prod. 2009, vol 72(30, pp 403-407.

[591]   Nigam N, et al. Induction of apoptosis by [6]-gingerol associated with the modulation of p53 and involvement of mitochondrial signaling pathway in B[a]P-induced mouse skin tumorigenesis. Cancer Chemother Pharmacol. 2010, vol 65(4), pp 687-696.

[592]   Siddaraju MN and Dharmesh SM. "Inhibition of gastric $H^+,K^+$-ATPase and *Helicobacter pylori* growth by phenolic antioxidants of *Zingiber officinale*." Molecular Nutrition Research. 2007, vol 51(3), pp 324-332.

[593]   Townsend EA, et al. "Effects of ginger and its constituents on airway smooth muscle relaxation and calcium regulation." American Journal of Respiratory Cell and Molecular Biology. 2013, vol 48(2), pp 157-163.

[594]   Zeng HL, et al. [Comparative protein analysis of K562 cell apoptosis induced by 6-gingerol]. Zhong Yao Cai. 2010, vol 33(5), p 753-758.

[595]   Chen Wei, et al. "The inhibition of quercetin and isorhamnetin on the proliferation of cultured human vascular smooth muscle cells." Chinese Journal of Cradiovascular Review. 2005-08.

[596]   Yi Wang, et al. "Simultaneous determination of quercetin, kaempferol and isorhamnetin accumulated human beast cancer cells, by high-performance liquid chromatography." Journal of Pharmaceutical and Biomedical Analysis. 2005, vol 39(1-2), pp 328-333.

[597]   Mursu J, et al. "Flavonoid intake and the risk of ischaemic stroke and CVD mortality
in middle-aged Finnish men: the Kuopio Ischaemic Heart Disease Risk Factor Study." British Journal of Nutrition. 2008, vol 100, pp 890-895.

[598]   Jaramillo S, et al. "The Flavonol Isorhamnetin Exhibits Cytotoxic Effects on Human Colon Cancer Cells." J Agric Food Chem. 2010, vol 58(20), pp 10869-10875.

[599]   Takako Yokozawa, et al. "Antioxidant Effects of Isorhamnetin 3,7-Di-*O*-β-d-glucopyranoside Isolated from Mustard Leaf (*Brassica juncea*) in Rats with Streptozotocin-Induced Diabetes." J Agric Food Chem. 2002, vol 50(19), pp 5490-5495.

[600]   Patel DK, et al. "Cataract: A major secondary complication of diabetes, its epidemiology and an overview on major medicinal plants screened for ant cataract activity." <u>Asian Pacific Journal of Tropical Disease.</u>  2011, p. 323-329.


[601]   Ma G, et al.. "The flavonoid component isorhamnetin in vitro inhibits proliferation and induces apoptosis in Eca-109 cells." <u>Chemico-Biological Interactions.</u>  2007, vol 167(2), pp 153-60.


[602]   Kannan M, et al. "HIV-1 reverse transcriptase inhibition by *Vitex negundo* L. leaf
extract and quantification of flavonoids in relation to anti-HIVActivity." <u>Journal of Cell and molecular Biology.</u> 2012, vol 10(2), pp 53-59.


[603]   Mursu J, et al. "Flavonoid intake and the risk of ischaemic stroke and CVD mortality
in middle-aged Finnish men: the Kuopio Ischaemic Heart Disease Risk Factor Study." <u>British Journal of Nutrition.</u> 2008, vol 100, pp 890-895.


[604]   Fu HY, et al. "Free Radical Scavenging and Leukemia Cell Growth Inhibitory Properties of Onion Powders Treated by Different Heating Processes." <u>Journal of Food Science.</u> 204, vol 69(1), pp SNQ50-SNQ54.


[605]   Lee HJ, et al. " Mitochondria-cytochrome C-caspase-9 cascade mediates isorhamnetin-induced apoptosis." Cancer Letters. 2008, vol 270(2), pp 342-353.


[606]   Frankenfeld CL, et al. "Dietary flavonoid intake and non-Hodgkin lymphoma risk." <u>Am J Clin Nutr.</u> 2008, vol 87(5), pp 1439-1445.


[607]   Bao-song Teng et al. "In vitro anti-tumor activity of isorhamnetin isolated from Hippophae rhamnoides L. against BEL-7402 cells." <u>Pharmacological Research.</u> 2006, vol 54(3),pp 186-194.


[608]   Jong-Eun Kim, et al. "Isorhamnetin Suppresses Skin Cancer through Direct Inhibition of MEK1 and PI3-K." <u>Cancer Prev Res.</u> 2011, vol 4, p 582.


[609]   Hollman PCH, et al. "Dietary Flavonol Intake May Lower Stroke Risk in Men and Women." <u>J Nutr.</u> 2010, vol 140(3), pp 600-604.

[610]  Bao-song Teng et al. "In vitro anti-tumor activity of isorhamnetin isolated from Hippophae rhamnoides L. against BEL-7402 cells." <u>Pharmacological Research.</u> 2006, vol 54(3),pp 186-194.

[611]  Huang XA, et al. Two new triterpenoids from Lysimachia heterogenea Klatt and evaluation of their cytotoxicity. Molecules. 2011, vol 16(9), pp 8076-8082.

[612]  Maheshwari DT, et al. Antioxidant and hepatoprotective activities of phenolic rich fraction of Seabuckthorn (Hippophae rhamnoides L.) leaves. Food Chem Toxicol. 2011, vol 49(9), pp 2422-2428.

[613]  Fu HY, et al. "Free Radical Scavenging and Leukemia Cell Growth Inhibitory Properties of Onion Powders Treated by Different Heating Processes." <u>Journal of Food Science.</u> 204, vol 69(1), pp SNQ50-SNQ54.

[614]  Ju-Hyun Gong, et al. "Kaempferol Suppresses Eosionphil Infiltration and Airway Inflammation in Airway Epithelial Cells and in Mice with Allergic Asthma." <u>J Nutr.</u> 2012, vol 142(1), pp 47-56.

[615]  JV Smith and Y Luo. "Elevation of oxidative free radicals in Alzheimer's disease models can be attenuated by Ginkgo biloba extract EGb 761." <u>Journal of Alzheimer's Disease.</u> 2003, vol 5(4), pp 287-300.

[616]  Kowalski J, et al. "Effect of apigenin, kaempferol and resveratrol on the expression of interleukin-1beta and tumor necrosis factor-alpha genes in J774.2 macrophages." <u>Pharmacological Reports.</u> 2005, vol 57(3), pp 390-394.

[617]  Kim ND, et al. "Chemopreventive and adjuvant therapeutic potential of pomegranate (Punica granatum) for human breast cancer." <u>Breast Cancer Research and Treatment.</u> 2002, vol 71(3), pp 203-217.

[618]  Kowalski J, et al. "Effect of apigenin, kaempferol and resveratrol on the expression of interleukin-1beta and tumor necrosis factor-alpha genes in J774.2 macrophages." <u>Pharmacological Reports.</u> 2005, vol 57(3), pp 390-394.

[619]  Neena Gandhi and Mahinda Wettasinghe.  Pyruvate Enviched Onion Extract. US Patent Application Publication No. US 2005/0037097 A1, Pub date Feb 17, 2005.

620   Kowalski J, et al. "Effect of apigenin, kaempferol and resveratrol on the expression of interleukin-1beta and tumor necrosis factor-alpha genes in J774.2 macrophages." <u>Pharmacological Reports.</u> 2005, vol 57(3), pp 390-394.

621   Yasushi Nakamura et al. Augmentation of differentiation and gap junction function by kaempferol in partially differentiated colon cancer cells. Carcinogenesis. 2005, vol 26 (3), pp 665-671.

622   Yun Jung Lee, et al. "Kaempferol protects HIT-T15 pancreatic beta cells from 2-deoxy-D-ribose-induced oxidative damage." <u>Phytotherapy Research.</u> 2010, vol 24(3), pp 419-423.

623   Milan stefek. "Natural Falconoid as Potential Multifunctional Agents in prevention of Diabetic Cataract." <u>Interdisciplinary Toxicology.</u> 2011, vol 4(2), pp 69-77.

624   Neena Gandhi and Mahinda Wettasinghe.  Pyruvate Enviched Onion Extract. US Patent Application Publication No. US 2005/0037097 A1, Pub date Feb 17, 2005.

625   Garcia-Closas R, et al. Intake of specific carotenoids and flavonoids and the risk of gastric cancer in Spain. Cancer Causes & Control. 1999, vol 10 (1), pp 71-75.

626   Kannan M, et al. "HIV-1 reverse transcriptase inhibition by *Vitex negundo* L. leaf extract and quantification of flavonoids in relation to anti-HIVActivity." <u>Journal of Cell and molecular Biology.</u> 2012, vol 10(2), pp 53-59.

627   Anke Esperester and Stephan nees. Use of falconoid compounds for the prophylaxis and therapy of ischemic or inflammatory heart and cardiovascular disease. US Patent Application Publication No. 2011/0053874 A1, Pub date March 3, 2011.

628   Mursu J, et al. "Flavonoid intake and the risk of ischaemic stroke and CVD mortality
in middle-aged Finnish men: the Kuopio Ischaemic Heart Disease Risk Factor Study." <u>British Journal of Nutrition.</u> 2008, vol 100, pp 890-895.

[629]  Garcia-Mediavilla V, et al. "The anti-inflammatory flavones quercetin and kaempferol cause inhibition of inducible nitric oxide synthase, cyclooxygenase-2 and reactive C-protein, and down-regulation of the nuclear factor kappaB pathway in Chang Liver cells." <u>European Journal of Pharmacology.</u> 2007, vol 557(2-3), pp 221-229.

[630]  Leung HWC, et al. "Kaempferol induces apoptosis in human lung non-small carcinoma cells accompanied by an induction of antioxidant enzymes." <u>Food and Chemical Toxicology.</u> 2007, vol 45(10), pp 2005-2013.

[631]  Hong-Xi Xu and Song F. Lee. "Activity of plant flavonoids against antibiotic-resistant bacteria." <u>Phytotherapy Research.</u> 2001(1), pp 39-43.

[632]  Frankenfeld CL, et al. "Dietary flavonoid intake and non-Hodgkin lymphoma risk." <u>Am J Clin Nutr.</u> 2008, vol 87(5), pp 1439-1445.

[633]  Ju Wan Kang, et al. Kaempferol and quercetin, components of Ginkgo biloba extract (EGb 761), induce caspase-3-dependent apoptosis in oral cavity cancer cells. Phytotherapy Research. 2010, vol 24 (S1), pp S77-S82.

[634]  Luo H et al. Kaempferol Inhibits Angiogenesis and VEGF Expression Through Both HIF Dependent and Independent Pathways in Human Ovarian Cancer Cells, Nutrition and Cancer. 2009, vol 61 (4).

[635]  Yuqing Zhang et al. *Ginkgo biloba* Extract Kaempferol Inhibits Cell Proliferation and Induces Apoptosis in Pancreatic Cancer Cells.  Journal of Surgical Research. 2008, vol 148 (1), pp 17-23.

[636]  Li S and Pu XP. Neuroprotective effect of kaempferol against a 1-methyl-4-phenyl-1,2,3,6-tetrahydropyridine-induced mouse model of Parkinson's disease. Biol Pharm Bull. 2011, vol 34(8), pp1291-1296.

[637]  Pantuck AJ, et al. "Phase II Study of Pomegranate Juice for Men with Rising Prostate-Specific Antigen following Surgery or Radiation for Prostate Cancer." <u>Clinical Cancer Res. 2006, vol 12, p 4018.</u> http://clincancerres.aacrjournals.org/content/12/13/4018.short

[638]  Garcia-Closas R, et al. Intake of specific carotenoids and flavonoids and the risk of gastric cancer in Spain. Cancer Causes & Control. 1999, vol 10 (1), pp 71-75.

[639]   Pamela Maher and Anne Hanneken. "Flavonoids Protect Retinal Ganglion Cells from Oxidative Stress–Induced Death." <u>Ophthalmol Vis Sci.</u> 2005, vol 46 (12), pp 4796-4803.

[640]   Hendra R, et al. "Flavonoid Analyses and Antimicrobial Activity of Various Parts of Phaleria macrocarpa (Scheff.) Boerl Fruit." <u>Int J Mol Sci.</u> 2011, vol 12(6), pp 3422-3431.

[641]  Li S and Pu XP. "Neuroprotective effect of kaempferol against a 1-methyl-4-phenyl-1,2,3,6-tetrahydropyridine-induced mouse model of Parkinson's disease." <u>Biol Pharm Bull</u>. 2011, vol 34(8), pp1291-1296.

[642]   Ono K, et al. "Preformed beta-amyloid fibrils are destabilized by coenzyme Q10 in vitro."
<u>Biochem and Biophys Res Commun</u>. 2005, vol. 330(1), pp 111-116.

[643]   Maggiolini M, et al. "The red wine phenolics piceatannol and myricetin act as agonists for estrogen receptor alpha in human breast cancer cells." <u>J Mol Endocrinol</u>. 2005, vol 35 (2), pp 269-281.

[644]   Hong-Xi Xu and Song F. Lee. "Activity of plant flavonoids against antibiotic-resistant bacteria." <u>Phytotherapy Research.</u> 2001(1), pp 39-43.

[645]   Mursu J, et al. "Flavonoid intake and the risk of ischaemic stroke and CVD mortality
in middle-aged Finnish men: the Kuopio Ischaemic Heart Disease Risk Factor Study." <u>British Journal of Nutrition.</u> 2008, vol 100, pp 890-895.

[646]   Nirmala P and Ramanathan M. "Effect of myricetin on 1,2 dimethylhydrazine induced rat colon carcinogenesis." <u>J Exp Ther Oncol</u>. 2011, vol 9(2), pp 101-108.

[647]   Ching-Huai Ko, et al.  "Myricetin inhibits matrix metalloproteinase 2 protein expression and enzyme activity in colorectal carcinoma cells." <u>Mol Cancer Ther.</u> 2005, vol 4, p 281.

[648]   I-Min Liu, et al. "Mediation of β-endorphin by myricetin to lower plasma glucose in streptozotocin-induced diabetic rats." <u>Journal of Ethnopharmacology.</u> 2006, vol104(1-2), pp 199-206.

[649]   Zhang Q, et al. "Cytotoxicity of flavones and flavonols to a human esophageal squamous cell carcinoma cell line (KYSE-510) by induction of G2/M arrest and apoptosis." <u>Toxicol In Vitro.</u> 2009, vol 23(5), pp 797-807.

[650]   Kannan M, et al. "HIV-1 reverse transcriptase inhibition by *Vitex negundo* L. leaf
extract and quantification of flavonoids in relation to anti-HIVActivity." <u>Journal of Cell and molecular Biology.</u> 2012, vol 10(2), pp 53-59.

[651]   Mursu J, et al. "Flavonoid intake and the risk of ischaemic stroke and CVD mortality
in middle-aged Finnish men: the Kuopio Ischaemic Heart Disease Risk Factor Study." <u>British Journal of Nutrition.</u> 2008, vol 100, pp 890-895.

[652]   Romanouskaya TV and Grinev VV. "Cytotoxic effect of flavonoids on leukemia cells and normal cells of human blood." <u>Bull Exp Biol Med</u>. 2009, vol 48(1), pp 57-59.

[653]   Zhang X, et al. "[Studies on mechanism of myricetin-induced apoptosis in human hepatocellular carcinoma HepG-2 cells]." <u>Zhongguo Zhong Yao Za Zhi.</u> 2010, vol 35(8), pp 1046-1050.

[654]   Jun Lu, et al. "Inhibition of Mammalian Thioredoxin Reductase by Some Flavonoids: Implications for Myricetin and Quercetin Anticancer Activity." <u>Cancer Research.</u> 2006, vol 66, p 410.

[655]   Frankenfeld CL, et al. "Dietary flavonoid intake and non-Hodgkin lymphoma risk." <u>Am J Clin Nutr.</u> 2008, vol 87(5), pp 1439-1445.

[656]   Kuo PL. "Myricetin inhibits the induction of anti-Fas IgM-, tumor necrosis factor-alpha- and interleukin-1beta-mediated apoptosis by Fas pathway inhibition in human osteoblastic cell line MG-63." <u>Life Sciences.</u> 2005, vol 77(23),pp 2964-2976.

[657]   Gates MA, et al. "Flavonoid intake and ovarian cancer risk in a population-based case-control study." <u>Int J Cancer</u>. 2009, vol 124(8), pp 1918-1925.

[658]   Phillips PA et al. "Myricetin induces pancreatic cancer cell death via the induction of apoptosis and inhibition of the phosphatidylinositol 3-kinase (PI3K) signaling pathway." <u>Cancer Lett</u>. 2011, vol 308(2), pp 181-188.

[659]  Ze Z-G, et al. "Myricetin reduces 6-hydroxydopamine-induced dopamine neuron degeneration in rats." Neuroreport. 2007, vol 18(11), pp 1181-1185.

[660]  Jankun J, et al. "Nutraceutical inhibitors of urokinase: potential applications in prostate cancer prevention and treatment." Oncol Rep. 2006, vol 16(2), pp 341-346.

[661]  Lee YS and Choi EM. "Myricetin inhibits IL-1beta-induced inflammatory mediators in SW982 human synovial sarcoma cells." Int Immunopharmacol. 2010, vol 10(7), pp 812--814.

[662]  Hong-Xi Xu and Song F. Lee. "Activity of plant flavonoids against antibiotic-resistant bacteria." Phytotherapy Research. 2001(1), pp 39-43.

[663]  Romanouskaya TV and Grinev VV. "Cytotoxic effect of flavonoids on leukemia cells and normal cells of human blood." Bull Exp Biol Med. 2009, vol 48(1), pp 57-59.

[664]  Nieman DC, et al. "Quercetin Reduces Illness but Not Immune Perturbations after Intensive Exercise." American College of Sports Medicine. 2007, pp 1561-1569.

[665]  Ansari MA, et al. "Protective Effect of Quercetin in Primary Neurons Against $A\beta(1-42)$: Relevance to Alzheimer's Disease." J Nutr Biochem. 2009, vol 20(4), pp 269-275.

[666]  CUI Yan, et al. "The Effect of Flavone on Vascular Endothelial Function of Female Patients with Angina Pectoris." Hebei Medicine. 2011, vol 11.

[667]  Priprem A, et al. "Anxiety and cognitive effects of quercetin liposomes in rats." Nan medicine: Nanotechnology, Biology and Medicine. 2008, vol 4 (1), pp 79-78.

[668]  Juzwiak S, et al. "Effect of quercetin on experimental hyperlipidemia and atherosclerosis in rabbits." Pharmacological Reports. 2005, vol 5, pp 604-609.

[669]  M Mamani-Matsuda et al. "Therapeutic and preventive properties of quercetin in experimental arthritis correlate with decreased macrophage inflammatory mediators." <u>Biochemical Pharmacology</u>. 2006, vol 72 (10), pp 1304-1310.

[670]  Garcia V, et al. "Dietary intake of flavonoids and asthma in adults." <u>ERJ</u>. 2005, vol 26 (3), pp 449-452.

[671]  Comalada M et al. "Immunomodulation In vivo quercitrin anti-inflammatory effect involves release of quercetin, which inhibits inflammation through down-regulation of the NF-κB pathway." <u>European journal of Immunology</u>. 2005, vol 35 (2), pp 584-592.

[672]  Choi JA et al. Induction of cell cycle arrest and apoptosis in human breast cancer cells by quercetin. International Journal of Oncology. 2001, vol 19 (4), pp 837-844.

[673]  Mursu J, et al. "Flavonoid intake and the risk of ischaemic stroke and CVD mortality in middle-aged Finnish men: the Kuopio Ischaemic Heart Disease Risk Factor Study." <u>British Journal of Nutrition.</u> 2008, vol 100, pp 890-895.

[674]  Sanderson J, et al. "Quercetin inhibits hydrogen peroxide-induced oxidation of the rat lens." <u>Free Radical Biology and Medicine.</u> 1999, vol 26(5-6), pp 639-645.

[675]  Maes M, et al. "Not in the mind of neurasthenic lazybones but in the cell nucleus: patients with chronic fatigue syndrome have increased production of nuclear factor kappa beta." <u>Endocrinology Letters.</u> 2007, vol 28(4), pp 456-462.

[676]  Garcia V, et al. Dietary intake of flavonoids and asthma in adults. ERJ. 2005, vol 26 (3), pp 449-452.

[677]  Shiu-Ming Kuo. Antiproliferative potency of structurally distinct dietary flavonoids on human colon cancer cells. Cancer Letters. 1996, vol 110 (1-2), pp 41-48.

[678]  Comalada M, et al. *In vivo* quercitrin anti-inflammatory effect involves release of quercetin, which inhibits inflammation through down-regulation of the NF-κB pathway. European Journal of Immunology. 2005, vol 35 (2), pp 584-592.

[679]  Adewole SO, et al. Protective effect of quartering on the morphology of pancreatic b-cells of streptozotocin-treated diabetic rats. Afr J Trad CAM. 2007, vol 4 (1), pp 64-74.

[680]  Valensi P, et al. A multicenter, double-blind, safety study of QR-333 for the treatment of symptomatic diabetic peripheral neuropathy: A preliminary report. Journal of Diabetes and its Complications. 2005, vol 19 (5), pp 247-253.

[681]  Lucas HJ, et al. "Fibromyalgia-new Concepts of  Pathogenesis and Treatment." International Journal of Immunopathology and Pharmacology. 2006, vol 19(1), pp 5-9.

[682]  Hamed Ghavimi, et al. Chamomile: An ancient pain remedy and a modern gout relief - A hypothesis. African journal of Pharmacy and Pharmacology. 2012, vol 6 (8), pp 508-511.

[683]  Kannan M, et al. "HIV-1 reverse transcriptase inhibition by *Vitex negundo* L. leaf extract and quantification of flavonoids in relation to anti-HIVActivity." Journal of Cell and molecular Biology. 2012, vol 10(2), pp 53-59.

[684]  Ramos FA, et al. "Antibacterial and Antioxidant Activities of Quercetin Oxidation Products from Yellow Onion (*Allium cepa*) skin." J Agric Food Chem. 2006, vol 54 (10), pp 3551-3557.

[685]  Comalada M et al, Immunomodulation *In vivo* quercitrin anti-inflammatory effect involves release of quercetin, which inhibits inflammation through down-regulation of the NF-κB pathway. Eauropean journal of Immunology. 2005, vol 35 (2), pp 584-592.

[686]  Heejung Kim et al. "Metabolic and Pharmacological Properties of Rutin, a Dietary Quercetin Glycoside, for Treatment of Inflammatory Bowel Disease." Pharmaceutical Research. 2005, vol 22 (9), pp 1499-1509.

[687]  Mursu J, et al. "Flavonoid intake and the risk of ischaemic stroke and CVD mortality
in middle-aged Finnish men: the Kuopio Ischaemic Heart Disease Risk Factor Study." British Journal of Nutrition. 2008, vol 100, pp 890-895.

[688]  Singh D, et al. "The effect of quercetin, a bioflavonoid on ischemia/reperfusion induced renal injury in rats." Archives of Medical Research. 2004, vol 35(6), pp 484-494.

[689]   Maes M, et al. "Normalization of leaky gut in chronic fatigue syndrome (CFS) is accompanied by a clinical improvement: effects of age, duration of illness and the translocation of LPS from gram-negative bacteria." <u>Neuroendocrinology Letters.</u> 2008, vol 29(6), pp 101-109.

[690]   Avci CB, et al. "Quercetin-induced apoptosis involves increased hTERT enzyme activity of leukemic cells." <u>Hematology.</u> 2011, vol 16(5), pp 303-307.

[691]   Pavanato A, et al. "Effects of Quercetin on Liver Damage in Rats with Carbon Tetrachloride-Induced Cirrhosis." <u>Digestive Diseases and Sciences.</u> 2003, vol 48(4), pp 824-829.

[692]   Murakami A, et al. "Multitargeted cancer prevention by quercetin." <u>Cancer Letters</u>. 2008, vol 269 (2), pp 315-325.

[693]   Hong-Xi Xu and Song F. Lee. "Activity of plant flavonoids against antibiotic-resistant bacteria." <u>Phytotherapy Research.</u> 2001(1), pp 39-43.

[694]   Frankenfeld CL, et al. "Dietary flavonoid intake and non-Hodgkin lymphoma risk." <u>Am J Clin Nutr.</u> 2008, vol 87(5), pp 1439-1445.

[695]   Mitsuyoshi Tsuji, et al. "Dietary quercetin inhibits bone loss without effect on the uterus in ovariectomized mice." <u>Journal of Bone and Mineral Metabolism.</u> 2009, vol 27(6), pp 673-381.

[696]   Haitao Luo et al. "Inhibition of Cell Growth and VEGF Expression in Ovarian Cancer Cells by Flavonoids." <u>Nutrition and Cancer</u>. 2008, vol 60 (6).

[697]   Adewole SO, et al. "Protective effect of quartering on the morphology of pancreatic b-cells of streptozotocin-treated diabetic rats." <u>Afr J Trad CAM</u>. 2007, vol 4 (1), pp 64-74.

[698]   Bureau G, et al. "Resveratrol and quercetin, two natural polyphenols, reduce apoptotic neuronal cell death induced by neuroinflammation." <u>Journal of Neuroscience Research.</u> 2008, vol 86(2), pp 403-410.

[699]   Vijayababu MR et al. "Quercetin downregulates matrix metalloproteinases 2 and 9 proteins expression in prostate cancer cells (PC-3)." <u>Molecular and Cellular Biochemistry.</u> 2006, vol 287 (1-2), pp 109-119.

[700] Calomme M, et al. "Inhibition of Bacterial Mutagenesis by Citrus Flavonoids." <u>Planta Med.</u> 1996, vol 62(3), pp 222-226.

[701] Garcia-Closas R, et al. "Intake of specific carotenoids and flavonoids and the risk of gastric cancer in Spain." <u>Cancer Causes & Control</u>. 1999, vol 10 (1), pp 71-75.

[702] Adewole SO, et al. Protective effect of quartering on the morphology of pancreatic b-cells of streptozotocin-treated diabetic rats. Afr J Trad CAM. 2007, vol 4 (1), pp 64-74.

[703] Juzwiak S, et al. "Effect of quercetin on experimental hyperlipidemia and atherosclerosis in rabbits." <u>Pharmacological Reports.</u> 2005, vol 5, pp 604-609.

[704] Comalada M et al, Immunomodulation In vivo quercitrin anti-inflammatory effect involves release of quercetin, which inhibits inflammation through down-regulation of the NF-$\kappa$B pathway. Eauropean journal of Immunology. 2005, vol 35 (2), pp 584-592.

[705] Lamson DW and Brignall MS. "Antioxidants and cancer, part 3: quercetin." <u>Alternative Medicine Review: a Journal of Clinical Therapeutic.</u> 2000, vol 5 (3), pp 196-208.

[706] Juzwiak S, et al. "Effect of quercetin on experimental hyperlipidemia and atherosclerosis in rabbits." <u>Pharmacological Reports.</u> 2005, vol 5, pp 604-609.

[707] Juzwiak S, et al. "Effect of quercetin on experimental hyperlipidemia and atherosclerosis in rabbits." <u>Pharmacological Reports.</u> 2005, vol 5, pp 604-609.

[708] Priprem A, et al. "Anxiety and cognitive effects of quercetin liposomes in rats." <u>Nan medicine: Nanotechnology, Biology and Medicine.</u> 2008, vol 4 (1), pp 79-78.

[709] Priprem A, et al. "Anxiety and cognitive effects of quercetin liposomes in rats." <u>Nan medicine: Nanotechnology, Biology and Medicine.</u> 2008, vol 4 (1), pp 79-78.

[710] Juzwiak S, et al. "Effect of quercetin on experimental hyperlipidemia and atherosclerosis in rabbits." <u>Pharmacological Reports.</u> 2005, vol 5, pp 604-609.

[711]   http://www.altmd.com/Articles/Bioflavonoids--Encyclopedia-of-Alternative-Medicine

[712]   Javed H, et al. "Rutin prevents cognitive impairments by ameliorating oxidative stress and neuroinflammation in rat model of sporadic dementia of Alzheimer type." Neuroscience. 2012, vol 210, pp 340-352.

[713]   F Fabjan. "Rutin, quercitrin and quercetin in buckwheat." Zbornik Biotehniske fakultete Univerze v Ljbljani. 2003, vol 81 (1), pp 151-159.

[714]   Guardia T et al. Anti-inflammatory properties of plant flavonoids. Effects of rutin, quercetin and hesperidin on adjuvant arthritis in rat. Il Farmaco, 2001 (9), pp 683-687.

[715]   Kim HB. Quantification and Varietal Variation of Rutin in Mulberry Fruits. Korean journal of Sericultural Science. 2004, vol 46 (1), pp 1-5.

[716]   Alia M, et al. "Influence of quercetin and rutin on growth and antioxidant defense system of a human hepatoma cell line (HepG2)." European Journal of Nutrition. 2006, vol 45(1), pp 19-28.

[717]   Yongmoon Han. "Rutin has therapeutic effect on septic arthritis caused by *Candida albicans*." International Immunopharmacology. 2009, vol 9(2), pp 207-211.

[718]   F Fabjan. Rutin, quercitrin and quercetin in buckwheat. Zbornik Biotehniske fakultete Univerze v Ljbljani. 2003, vol 81 (1), pp 151-159.

[719]   Ihme N, et al. "Leg oedema protection from a buckwheat herb tea in patients with chronic venous insufficiency: a single-centre, randomised, double-blind, placebo-controlled clinical trial." European Journal of Clinical Pharmacology. 1996, vol 50(6), pp 443-447.

[720]   Ki Han Kwon, et al. "Dietary rutin, but not its aglycone quercetin, ameliorates dextran sulfate sodium-induced experimental colitis in mice: attenuation of pro-inflammatory gene expression." Biochemical Pharmacology. 2005, vol 69(3), pp 395-406.

[721]  Levitan BA. "Clinical Observations on the Effects of Injectable Rutin, Esculin, Adrenoxyl, and Vitamin E on the Capillary Fragility of Diabetic Retinopathy." <u>American Journal of the Medical Sciences.</u> 1951, vol 221(2), pp 185-190.

[722]  So Youn Mok et al. "Inhibition of Aldose Reductase on Rant Lens by Tartary Buckwheat." <u>Natural Product Sciences</u>. 2011, vol 17 (3), pp 230-233.

Fernandes AA, et al. "Influence of rutin treatment on biochemical alterations in experimental diabetes." <u>Biomed Pharmacother</u>. 2010, vol 64(3), pp 214-219.

[723]  Chin-Lin Hsu, et al. "Phenolic Compounds Rutin and *o*-Coumaric Acid Ameliorate Obesity Induced by High-Fat Diet in Rats." <u>J Agric Food Chem.</u> 2009, vol 57(2), pp 425-431.

[724]  La Casa, C, et al. "Evidence for protective and antioxidant properties of rutin, a natural flavone, against ethanol induced gastric lesions." <u>Journal of Ethnopharmacology.</u> 2000, vol 71(1-2), pp 45-53.

[725]  Wu CH, et al. "Rutin inhibits oleic acid induced lipid accumulation via reducing lipogenesis and oxidative stress in hepatocarcinoma cells." <u>J Food Sci</u>. 2011, vol 76(2), pp T65-72.

[726]  Pescosolido N and Librando A. "Oral administration of an association of forskolin, rutin and vitamins B1 and B2 potentiates the hypotonising effects of pharmacological treatments in POAG patients."<u>La Clinica Terapeutica.</u> 2010, vol 161(3), pp e81-e85.

[727]  Mohammad Arif Dar and Nahida Tabassum. "Rutin- potent natural thrombolytic agent."
<u>International Current Pharmaceutical Journal.</u> 2012, vol 1 (12).

[728]  Kim HB. "Quantification and Varietal Variation of Rutin in Mulberry Fruits." <u>Korean Journal of Sericultural Science.</u> 2004, vol 46 (1), pp 1-5.

[729]  Chin-Lin Hsu, et al. "Phenolic Compounds Rutin and *o*-Coumaric Acid Ameliorate Obesity Induced by High-Fat Diet in Rats." <u>J Agric Food Chem.</u> 2009, vol 57(2), pp 425-431.

[730]  Borissova P et al. Antiinflammatory effect of flavonoids in the natural juice from Aronia melanocarpa, rutin and rutin-magnesium complex on an experimental model of inflammation induced by histamine and serotonin. Acta Physiologica et Pharmacologica Bulgarica. 2004, vol 20 (1), pp 25-30.

[731]  Kanashiro A, et al. "Modulatory effects of rutin on biochemical and hematological parameters in hypercholesterolemic Golden Syrian hamsters." Anais da Academia Brasileira de Ciencias. 2009, vol 81(1).

[732]  Henrique Fernandes AA, et al. "Influence of rutin treatment on biochemical alterations in experimental diabetes." Biomedicine & Pharmacotherapy. 2010, vol 64(3), pp 214-219.

[733]  Ki Han Kwon, et al. "Dietary rutin, but not its aglycone quercetin, ameliorates dextran sulfate sodium-induced experimental colitis in mice: attenuation of pro-inflammatory gene expression." Biochemical Pharmacology. 2005, vol 69(3), pp 395-406.

[734]  Khan MM, et al. Rutin protects the neural damage induced by transient focal ischemia in rats. Brain Res. 2009, vol 1292, pp 123-135.

[735]  Nassiri-Asl M, et al. "The effects of rutin on a passive avoidance test in rats." Progress in Neuro-Psychopharmacology and Biological Psychiatry. 2010, vol 34(1), pp 204-207.

[736]  Martinez CC, et al. "Treatment of metastatic melanoma B16F10 by the flavonoids tangeretin, rutin, and diosmin." J Agric Food Chem. 2005, vol 53(17), pp 6791-6797.

[737]  Chin-Lin Hsu, et al. "Phenolic Compounds Rutin and o-Coumaric Acid Ameliorate Obesity Induced by High-Fat Diet in Rats." J Agric Food Chem. 2009, vol 57(2), pp 425-431.

[738]  Nianzeng Xing, et al. Quercetin inhibits the expression and function of the androgen receptor in LNCaP prostate cancer cells. Carcinogenesis. 2001, vol 22 (3), pp 409-411.

[739]  Patil SL et  al. Evaluation of the Radioprotective action of mice exposed to Gamma-radiation. International Journal of Biological & Pharmaceutical Research. 2012, vol 3 (1), pp 12-8.

[740]   Devi VS, et al. "RADIATION SICKNESS-NEED TO UNDERSTAND, AWARE AND ROLE OF HERBS IN THE MANAGEMENT ITS IMPACT ON HUMANS-AN OVERVIEW." INTERNATIONAL Journal of Ayurvedic. 2013. Interscience.org.uk

Patil SL, et al. "EVALUATION OF THE RADIOPROTECTIVE ACTION OF RUTIN IN MICE EXPOSED TO GAMMA-RADIATION." International Journal of Biological & Pharmaceutical Research. 2013, vol 3(1), pp 12-18.

[741]   Guardia T, et al. "Anti-inflammatory properties of plant flavonoids. Effects of rutin, quercetin and hesperidin on adjuvant arthritis in rat." Il Farmaco. 2001, vol 56(9), pp 683-687.

[742]   Yongmoon Han. "Rutin has therapeutic effect on septic arthritis caused by *Candida albicans*." International Immunopharmacology. 2009, vol 9(2), pp 207-211.

[743]   Javed H, et al. "Rutin prevents cognitive impairments by ameliorating oxidative stress and neuroinflammation in rat model of sporadic dementia of Alzheimer type." Neuroscience. 2012, vol 210, pp 340-352.

[744]   Mohammad Arif Dar and Nahida Tabassum. Rutin- potent natural thrombolytic agent
International Current Pharmaceutical Journal. 2012, vol 1 (12).

[745]   Bishnoi M, et al. "Protective effect of rutin, a polyphenolic flavonoid against haloperidol-induced orofacial dyskinesia and associated behavioural, biochemical and neurochemical changes." Fundamental & Clinical Pharmacology. 2007, vol 21(5), pp 521-539.

[746]   Mohammad Arif Dar and Nahida Tabassum. "Rutin- potent natural thrombolytic agent."
International Current Pharmaceutical Journal. 2012, vol 1 (12).

[747]   Kanashiro A, et al. "Modulatory effects of rutin on biochemical and hematological parameters in hypercholesterolemic Golden Syrian hamsters." Anais da Academia Brasileira de Ciencias. 2009, vol 81(1).

[748]  Ushida Y, et al. "Endothelium-dependent vasorelaxation effect of rutin-free tartary buckwheat extract in isolated rat thoracic aorta." Journal of Nutritional Biochemistry. 2008, vol 19(10), pp 700-707.

[749]  Kim HB. "Quantification and Varietal Variation of Rutin in Mulberry Fruits." Korean journal of Sericultural Science. 2004, vol 46 (1), pp 1-5.

[750]  Ibid.

[751]  Mohammad Arif Dar and Nahida Tabassum. "Rutin- potent natural thrombolytic agent."
International Current Pharmaceutical Journal. 2012, vol 1 (12).

[752]  Yongmoon Han. "Rutin has therapeutic effect on septic arthritis caused by *Candida albicans*." International Immunopharmacology. 2009, vol 9(2), pp 207-211.

[753]  Borissova P et al. Antiinflammatory effect of flavonoids in the natural juice from Aronia melanocarpa, rutin and rutin-magnesium complex on an experimental model of inflammation induced by histamine and serotonin. Acta Physiologica et Pharmacologica Bulgarica. 2004, vol 20 (1), pp 25-30.

[754]  Yongmoon Han. "Rutin has therapeutic effect on septic arthritis caused by *Candida albicans*." International Immunopharmacology. 2009, vol 9(2), pp 207-211.

[755]  Nassiri-Asl M, et al. "Anticonvulsive effects of intracerebroventricular administration of rutin in rats." Progress in Neuro-Psychopharmacology and Biological Psychiatry. 2008, vol 32(4), pp 989-993,

[756]  Kim HB. Quantification and Varietal Variation of Rutin in Mulberry Fruits. Korean journal of Sericultural Science. 2004, vol 46 (1), pp 1-5.

[757]  Yongmoon Han. "Rutin has therapeutic effect on septic arthritis caused by *Candida albicans*." International Immunopharmacology. 2009, vol 9(2), pp 207-211.

[758]  Kim JM and Yun-Choi HS. Anti-platelet effects of flavonoids and flavonoid-glycosides from Sophora japonica. Arch Pharm Res. 2008, vol 31(7), pp 886-890.

759  Xue Tian, et al. Study on the electrochemical behavior of anticancer herbal drug rutin and its interaction with DNA. Journal of Electroanalytical Chemistry. 2008, vol 621 (1), pp 1-6.

760  Khan MM, et al. Rutin protects the neural damage induced by transient focal ischemia in rats. Brain Res. 2009, vol 1292, pp 123-135.

761  Patil SL et al. Evaluation of the Radioprotective action of mice exposed to Gamma-radiation. International Journal of Biological & Pharmaceutical Research. 2012, vol 3 (1), pp 12-8.

762  Kim HB. "Quantification and Varietal Variation of Rutin in Mulberry Fruits." Korean Journal of Sericultural Science. 2004, vol 46 (1), pp 1-5.

763  Bonnie Prescott. "Flavonoid compound can prevent blood clots." Harvard Science. may 9, 2012.

764  Guardia T, et al. "Anti-inflammatory properties of plant flavonoids. Effects of rutin, quercetin and hesperidin on adjuvant arthritis in rat." Il Farmaco. 2001, vol 56(9), pp 683-687.

765  Sang Keun Ha, et al. "Apigenin inhibits the production of NO and $PGE_2$ in microglia and inhibits neuronal cell death in a middle cerebral artery occlusion-induced focal ischemia mice model." Neurochemistry International. 2008, vol 52(4-5), pp 878-886.

766  S Kimar and A Sharma. "Apigenin: The Anxiolytic Constituent of Turnera aphrodisiaca." Pharmaceutical Biology. 2006, vol 44(2), pp 84-90.

767  Sanjeev Shukla and Sanjay Gupta. "Apigenin: A Promising Molecule for Cancer Prevention." Pharm Res. 2010, vol 27(6), pp 962-978.

768  Sanjeev Shukla and Sanjay Gupta. "Apigenin: A Promising Molecule for Cancer Prevention." Pharm Res. 2010, vol 27(6), pp 962-978.

769  Sang Keun Ha, et al. "Apigenin inhibits the production of NO and $PGE_2$ in microglia and inhibits neuronal cell death in a middle cerebral artery occlusion-induced focal ischemia mice model." Neurochemistry International. 2008, vol 52(4-5), pp 878-886.

[770] Leonardi T, et al. "Apigenin and naringenin suppress colon carcinogenesis through the aberrant crypt stage in azoxymethane-treated rats." <u>Exp Biol Med (Maywood).</u> 2010, vol 235(6), pp 710-717.

[771] Sanjeev Shukla and Sanjay Gupta. "Apigenin: A Promising Molecule for Cancer Prevention." <u>Pharm Res.</u> 2010, vol 27(6), pp 962-978.

[772] Sanjeev Shukla and Sanjay Gupta. "Apigenin: A Promising Molecule for Cancer Prevention." Pharm Res. 2010, vol 27(6), pp 962-978.

[773] Zhao G, et al. "Functional activation of monoamine transporters by luteolin and apigenin isolated from the fruit of Perilla frutescens (L.) Britt." <u>Neurochem Int.</u> 2010, vol 56(1), pp 168-176.

[774] Philippe Taupir. "Apigenin and related compounds stimulate adult neurogenesis Mars, Inc., the Salk Institute for Biological Studies: WO2008147483." <u>Expert Opinion on Therapeutic Patents.</u> 2009, vol 19(4), pp 523-427.

[775] Ruela-de-Sousa RR, et al. "Cytotoxicity of apigenin on leukemia cell lines: implications for prevention and therapy." <u>Cell Death Dis.</u> 2010, vol 1(1), pp e19.

[776] Ren HY and Tang XW. "[Anti-proliferation and chemo-sensitization effects of apigenin on human lung cancer cells]." <u>Zhejiang Da Xue Xue Bao Yi Xue Ban.</u> 2011, vol 40(5), pp 508-514.

[777] Hussain AR, et al. "Apigenin induces apoptosis *via* downregulation of S-phase kinase-associated protein 2-mediated induction of p27Kip1 in primary effusion lymphoma cells." <u>Cell Proliferation.</u> 2010, vol 43(2), pp 170-183.

[778] Ebrahimi A and Schluesener H. "Natural polyphenols against neurodegenerative disorders: Potentials and pitfalls." 2012, vol 11(2), pp 329-345.

[779] Sanjeev Shukla and Sanjay Gupta. "Apigenin: A Promising Molecule for Cancer Prevention." Pharm Res. 2010, vol 27(6), pp 962-978.

[780] Frankenfeld CL, et al. "Dietary flavonoid intake and non-Hodgkin lymphoma risk." <u>Am J Clin Nutr.</u> 2008, vol 87(5), pp 1439-1445.

781   Hyeon-Jong Myoung, et al. "Apigenin isolated from the seeds of Perilla frutescens britton var crispa (Benth.) inhibits food intake in C57BL/6J mice." Archives of Pharmacal Research. 2010, vol 33(11), pp 1741-1746.

782   Silvan S, et al. "Chemopreventive potential of apigenin in 7,12-dimethylbenz(a)anthracene induced experimental oral carcinogenesis." Eur J Pharmacol. 2011, vol 670(2-3), pp 571-577.

783   Sang Keun Ha, et al. "Apigenin inhibits the production of NO and $PGE_2$ in microglia and inhibits neuronal cell death in a middle cerebral artery occlusion-induced focal ischemia mice model." Neurochemistry International. 2008, vol 52(4-5), pp 878-886.

784   Nakazaki E, et al. "Proteomic study of granulocytic differentiation induced by apigenin 7-glucoside in human promyelocytic leukemia HL-60 cells." Eur J Nutr. 2013, vol 52(1), pp 25-35.

785   Sanjeev Shukla and Sanjay Gupta. "Apigenin: A Promising Molecule for Cancer Prevention." Pharm Res. 2010, vol 27(6), pp 962-978.

786   Srikumar Chakravarthi, et al. "Apoptosis and expression of bcl-2 in cyclosporine induced
renal damage and its reversal by beneficial effects of 4', 5', 7'- trihydroxyflavone." Journal of Analytical Bio-Science. 2009, vol 32(4), pp 320-327.

787   Wang Y, et al. "Flavone C-glycosides from the leaves of Lophatherum gracile and their in vitro antiviral activity." Planta Med. 2012, vol 78(1), pp 46-51.

788   Masoumeh Kheirabadi, et al. "Evaluation of the Anticonvulsant Activities of Rosa dmascena on the PTZ Induced Seizures in Wistar Rats." Journal of Biological Sciences. 2008, vol 8(2), pp 426-430.

789   Sanjeev Shukla and Sanjay Gupta. "Apigenin: A Promising Molecule for Cancer Prevention." Pharm Res. 2010, vol 27(6), pp 962-978.

790   Philippe Taupin. "Apigenin and related compounds stimulate adult neurogenesis." Informa Healthcare. Mars, Inc., the Salk Institute for Biological Studies: WO2008147483. 2009, vol 19(4), pp 523-527.

[791]  Hui Zhou. "Mechanism of CYP2C9 Inhibition by Flavones and Flavonols." DMD. 2009, vol 37(3), p 629.

[792]  Sanjeev Shukla and Sanjay Gupta. "Apigenin: A Promising Molecule for Cancer Prevention." Pharm Res. 2010, vol 27(6), pp 962-978.

[793]  Chaves DS, et al. "Phenolic chemical composition of Petroselinum crispum extract and its effect on haemostasis." Nat Prod Commun. 2011, vol 6(7), pp 961-964.

[794]  Wang Y, et al. "Flavone C-glycosides from the leaves of Lophatherum gracile and their in vitro antiviral activity." Planta Med. 2012, vol 78(1), pp 46-51.

[795]  S Kimar and A Sharma. "Apigenin: The Anxiolytic Constituent of Turnera aphrodisiaca." Pharmaceutical Biology. 2006, vol 44(2), pp 84-90.

[796]  Seo YJ, et al. "Apoptotic effects of genistein, biochanin-A and apigenin on LNCaP and PC-3 cells by p21 through transcriptional inhibition of polo-like kinase-1." J Korean Med Sci. 2011, vol 26(11), pp 1489-1494.

[797]  Wang Y, et al. "Flavone C-glycosides from the leaves of Lophatherum gracile and their in vitro antiviral activity." Planta Med. 2012, vol 78(1), pp 46-51.

[798]  Perez Gutierrez RM, et al. "Effect of flavonoids from Prosthechea michuacana on carbon tetrachloride induced acute hepatotoxicity in mice." Pharm Biol. 2011, vol 49(11), 1121-1127.

[799]  Losi G, et al. "Apigenin modulates GABAergic and glutamatergic transmission in cultured cortical neurons." European Journal of Pharmacology. 2004, vol 502(1-2), pp 41-46.

[800]  Masoumeh Kheirabadi, et al. "Evaluation of the Anticonvulsant Activities of Rosa dmascena on the PTZ Induced Seizures in Wistar Rats." Journal of Biological Sciences. 2008, vol 8(2), pp 426-430.

[801]  Zhao G, et al. "Functional activation of monoamine transporters by luteolin and apigenin isolated from the fruit of Perilla frutescens (L.) Britt." Neurochem Int. 2010, vol 56(1), pp 168-176.

[802] Chaves DS, et al. "Phenolic chemical composition of Petroselinum crispum extract and its effect on haemostasis." <u>Nat Prod Commun.</u> 2011, vol 6(7), pp 961-964.

[803] Masoumeh Kheirabadi, et al. "Evaluation of the Anticonvulsant Activities of Rosa dmascena on the PTZ Induced Seizures in Wistar Rats." <u>Journal of Biological Sciences.</u> 2008, vol 8(2), pp 426-430.

[804] Agarwal A and S Partners. "(WO2007141807) A SYNERGISTIC HERBAL COMPOSITION FROM BACOPA SPECIES FOR MANAGEMENT OF NEURODEGENERATIVE DISORDERS AND A PROCESS OF PREPARATION THEREOF ." <u>Patentscope.</u> Pub. Date 13.12.2007.

[805] Wruck CJ, et al. "Luteolin protects rat PC 12 and C6 cells against MPP+ induced toxicity via an ERK dependent Keapl-Nrf2-ARE pathway." <u>Neuropsychiatric Disorders An Integrative Approach.</u> 2007, vol 72, pp 57-67.

[806] Theoharides TC, et al. "A case series of a luteolin formulation (NeuroProtek®) in children with autism spectrum disorders." <u>Int J Immunopathol Pharmacol.</u> 2012, vol 25(2), pp 317-323.

[807] Kayoko Shimol, et al. "Metabolic fate of luteolin and its functional activity at focal site." <u>BioFactors.</u> 2000, vol 12(1-4), pp 181-186.

[808] Theoharides TC, et al. "A case series of a luteolin formulation (NeuroProtek®) in children with autism spectrum disorders." <u>Int J Immunopathol Pharmacol.</u> 2012, vol 25(2), pp 317-323.

[809] Pereira AP, et al. "Phenolic Compounds and Antimicrobial Activity of Olive (*Olea europaea* L. *Cv.* Cobrançosa) Leaves." <u>Molecules.</u> 2007, vol 12(5), pp 1153-1162.

[810] Ibid.

[811] Tae-Ho Kim, et al. "The effects of luteolin on osteoclast differentiation, function in vitro and ovariectomy-induced bone loss." <u>Journal of Nutritional Biochemistry.</u> 2011, vol 22(1), pp 8-15.

[812] Kayoko Shimol, et al. "Metabolic fate of luteolin and its functional activity at focal site." <u>BioFactors.</u> 2000, vol 12(1-4), pp 181-186.

[813]   Kim ND, et al. "Chemopreventive and adjuvant therapeutic potential of pomegranate (Punica granatum) for human breast cancer." <u>Breast Cancer Research and Treatment.</u> 2002, vol 71(3), pp 203-217.

[814]   Seelinger F, et al. "Anti-carcinogenic Effects of the Flavonoid Luteolin." <u>Molecules.</u> 2008, vol 13(10), pp 2628-2651.

[815]   Pereira AP, et al. "Phenolic Compounds and Antimicrobial Activity of Olive (*Olea europaea* L. *Cv.* Cobrançosa) Leaves." <u>Molecules.</u> 2007, vol 12(5), pp 1153-1162.

[816]   Agarwal A and S Partners. "(WO2007141807) A SYNERGISTIC HERBAL COMPOSITION FROM BACOPA SPECIES FOR MANAGEMENT OF NEURODEGENERATIVE DISORDERS AND A PROCESS OF PREPARATION THEREOF ." <u>Patentscope.</u> Pub. Date 13.12.2007.

[817]   Do Y Lim, et al. "Induction of cell cycle arrest and apoptosis in HT-29 human colon cancer cells by the dietary compound luteolin." <u>AJP.</u> 2006, vol 292(1), pp G66-G75.

[818]   Pereira AP, et al. "Phenolic Compounds and Antimicrobial Activity of Olive (*Olea europaea* L. *Cv.* Cobrançosa) Leaves." <u>Molecules.</u> 2007, vol 12(5), pp 1153-1162.

[819]   Pereira AP, et al. "Phenolic Compounds and Antimicrobial Activity of Olive (*Olea europaea* L. *Cv.* Cobrançosa) Leaves." <u>Molecules.</u> 2007, vol 12(5), pp 1153-1162.

[820]   Begum N, et al. "Apigenin protects gamma-radiation induced oxidative stress, hematological changes and animal survival in whole body irradiated Swiss albino mice." <u>International Journal of Nutrition, Pharmacology, Neurological Diseases.</u> 2012, vol 2(1), pp 45-52.

[821]   Ming-Chih Yu, et al. "Luteolin, a non-selective competitive inhibitor of phosphodiesterases 1–5, displaced [$^3$H]-rolipram from high-affinity rolipram binding sites and reversed xylazine/ketamine-induced anesthesia." <u>Euro J of Pharm</u>. 2010, vol 627(1-3), pp 1-3.

822   Young Sil Min, et al. "The effect of luteolin-7-O-β-d-glucuronopyranoside on gastritis and esophagitis in rats." <u>Archives of Pharmacol Research.</u> 2006, vol 29(6), pp 484-489.

823   Kannan M, et al. "HIV-1 reverse transcriptase inhibition by *Vitex negundo* L. leaf
extract and quantification of flavonoids in relation to anti-HIVActivity." <u>Journal of Cell and molecular Biology.</u> 2012, vol 10(2), pp 53-59.

824   Zhao G, et al. "Functional activation of monoamine transporters by luteolin and apigenin isolated from the fruit of Perilla frutescens (L.) Britt." <u>Neurochem Int.</u> 2010, vol 56(1), pp 168-176.

825   Pereira AP, et al. "Phenolic Compounds and Antimicrobial Activity of Olive (*Olea europaea* L. *Cv.* Cobrançosa) Leaves." <u>Molecules.</u> 2007, vol 12(5), pp 1153-1162.

826   Agarwal A and S Partners. "(WO2007141807) A SYNERGISTIC HERBAL COMPOSITION FROM BACOPA SPECIES FOR MANAGEMENT OF NEURODEGENERATIVE DISORDERS AND A PROCESS OF PREPARATION THEREOF ." <u>Patentscope.</u> Pub. Date 13.12.2007.

827   Ibid.

828   Asadi S, et al. "Luteolin and thiosalicylate inhibit HgCl(2) and thimerosal-induced VEGF release from human mast cells." <u>Int J Immunopathol Pharmacol.</u> 2010, vol 23(4), pp 1015-1020.

829   Theoharides TC. "Luteolin as a therapeutic option for multiple sclerosis." <u>J Neuroinflammation</u>. 2009 Oct 13, vol 6, p 29.

830   Ebrahimi A and Schluesener H. "Natural polyphenols against neurodegenerative disorders: Potentials and pitfalls." 2012, vol 11(2), pp 329-345.

831   Frankenfeld CL, et al. "Dietary flavonoid intake and non-Hodgkin lymphoma risk." <u>Am J Clin Nutr.</u> 2008, vol 87(5), pp 1439-1445.

832   Tae-Ho Kim, et al. "The effects of luteolin on osteoclast differentiation, function in vitro and ovariectomy-induced bone loss." <u>Journal of Nutritional Biochemistry.</u> 2011, vol 22(1), pp 8-15.

[833]   Haitao Luo, et al. "Inhibition of Cell Growth and VEGF Expression in Ovarian Cancer Cells by Flavonoids." <u>Nutrition and Cancer.</u> 2008, vol 60(6), pp 800-809.

[834]   Lee SW, et al. "Inhibitory Effect of Flavonoid Luteolin on 6-Hydroxydopamine Cytotoxicity via Suppression of Apoptosis-Related Protein Activation." <u>J Korean Neurol Assoc.</u> 2012, vol 30(4), pp 284-292.

[835]   Tsui KH, et al. "Upregulation of prostate-derived Ets factor by luteolin causes inhibition of cell proliferation and cell invasion in prostate carcinoma cells." <u>Int J Cancer.</u> 2010, vol 130(12), pp 2812-2823.

[836]   Pereira AP, et al. "Phenolic Compounds and Antimicrobial Activity of Olive (*Olea europaea* L. *Cv.* Cobrançosa) Leaves." <u>Molecules.</u> 2007, vol 12(5), pp 1153-1162.

[837]   Young Sil Min, et al. "The effect of luteolin-7-O-$\beta$-d-glucuronopyranoside on gastritis and esophagitis in rats." <u>Archives of Pharmacol Research.</u> 2006, vol 29(6), pp 484-489.

[838]   Kayoko Shimol, et al. "Metabolic fate of luteolin and its functional activity at focal site." <u>BioFactors.</u> 2000, vol 12(1-4), pp 181-186.

[839]   Seelinger F, et al. "Anti-carcinogenic Effects of the Flavonoid Luteolin." <u>Molecules.</u> 2008, vol 13(10), pp 2628-2651.

[840]   Pereira AP, et al. "Phenolic Compounds and Antimicrobial Activity of Olive (*Olea europaea* L. *Cv.* Cobrançosa) Leaves." <u>Molecules.</u> 2007, vol 12(5), pp 1153-1162.

[841]   Wolfle U, et al. "UVB-induced DNA damage, generation of reactive oxygen species, and inflammation are effectively attenuated by the flavonoid luteolin *in vitro* and *in vivo*." <u>Free Radical Biology and Medicine.</u> 2011, vol 50(9), pp 1081-1093.

[842]   Chung JG, et al. "Inhibitory actions of luteolin on the growth and arylamine *N*-acetyltransferase activity in strains of *Helicobacter pylori* from ulcer patients." <u>Toxicology in Vitro.</u> 2001, vol 15(3) ppp 191-198.

[843]  Chowdhury AR, et al.. "Luteolin, an emerging anti-cancer flavonoid, poisons eukaryotic DNA topoisomerase I." Biochem J.  2002, vol 366(Pt 2), pp 653-661.

[844]  Pereira AP, et al. "Phenolic Compounds and Antimicrobial Activity of Olive (*Olea europaea* L. *Cv.* Cobrançosa) Leaves." Molecules. 2007, vol 12(5), pp 1153-1162.

[845]  Ibid.

[846]  Ibid.

[847]  Seelinger F, et al. "Anti-carcinogenic Effects of the Flavonoid Luteolin." Molecules. 2008, vol 13(10), pp 2628-2651.

[848]  Ming-Chih Yu, et al. "Luteolin, a non-selective competitive inhibitor of phosphodiesterases 1–5, displaced [$^3$H]-rolipram from high-affinity rolipram binding sites and reversed xylazine/ketamine-induced anesthesia." Euro J of Pharm. 2010, vol 627(1-3), pp 1-3.

[849]  Agarwal A and S Partners. "(WO2007141807) A SYNERGISTIC HERBAL COMPOSITION FROM BACOPA SPECIES FOR MANAGEMENT OF NEURODEGENERATIVE DISORDERS AND A PROCESS OF PREPARATION THEREOF ." Patentscope. Pub. Date 13.12.2007.

[850]  Zhao G, et al. "Functional activation of monoamine transporters by luteolin and apigenin isolated from the fruit of Perilla frutescens (L.) Britt." Neurochem Int. 2010, vol 56(1), pp 168-176.

[851]  Asadi S, et al. "Luteolin and thiosalicylate inhibit HgCl(2) and thimerosal-induced VEGF release from human mast cells." Int J Immunopathol Pharmacol. 2010, vol 23(4), pp 1015-1020.

[852]  Ebrahimi A and Schluesener H. "Natural polyphenols against neurodegenerative disorders: Potentials and pitfalls." 2012, vol 11(2), pp 329-345.

[853]  Juhee Seo, et al. "Tangeretin, a citrus flavonoid, inhibits PGDF-BB-induced proliferation and migration of aortic smooth muscle cells by blocking AKT activation." European journal of Pharmacology. 2011, vol 673(1-3), pp 56-64.

854   Alleva LM, et al. "Current work and future possibilities for the management of severe influenza: using immunomodulatory agents that target the host response." <u>Future Virology.</u> 2011, vol 6(7), pp 843-854. http://www.futuremedicine.com/doi/abs/10.2217/fvl.11.51

855   Morley KL, et al. "Tangeretin and nobiletin induce G1 cell cycle arrest but not apoptosis in human breast and colon cancer cells." <u>Cancer Lett</u>. 2007, vol 251(1), pp 168-178.

856   Juhee Seo, et al. "Tangeretin, a citrus flavonoid, inhibits PGDF-BB-induced proliferation and migration of aortic smooth muscle cells by blocking AKT activation." <u>European journal of Pharmacology.</u> 2011, vol 673(1-3), pp 56-64.

857   Morley KL, et al. "Tangeretin and nobiletin induce G1 cell cycle arrest but not apoptosis in human breast and colon cancer cells." <u>Cancer Lett</u>. 2007, vol 251(1), pp 168-178.

858   Williams RJ and Spencer JPE. "Flavonoids, cognition, and dementia: Actions, mechanisms, and potential therapeutic utility for Alzheimer disease." <u>Free Radical Biology and Medicine.</u> 2012, vol 52(1), pp 35-45.

859   Veljkovic V, et al. "Simple criterion for selection of flavonoid compounds with anti-HIV activity." <u>Bioorganic & Medicinal Chemistry.</u> 2007, vol 17(5), pp 1226-1232.

860   Cintron JR and Abcarian H. "Benign Anorectal: Hemorrhoids." <u>ASCRS Textbook of Colon and Rectal Surgery.</u> 2007, pp 156-177.

861   Alleva LM, et al. "Current work and future possibilities for the management of severe influenza: using immunomodulatory agents that target the host response." <u>Future Virology.</u> 2011, vol 6(7), pp 843-854.

862   Fan K, et al. "Chemopreventive effects of orange peel extract (OPE). I: OPE inhibits intestinal tumor growth in ApcMin/+ mice." <u>J Med Food.</u> 2007, vol 10(1), pp 11-17.

863   Bracke ME, et al. "The flavonoid tangeretin inhibits invasion of MO4 mouse cells into embryonic chick heart in vitro." <u>Clinical & Experimental Metastasis.</u> 1989, vol 7(3), pp 283-300.

[864]  Hirano T, et al. "Citrus flavone tangeretin inhibits leukaemic HL-60 cell growth partially through induction of apoptosis with less cytotoxicity on normal lymphocytes." Br J Cancer. 1995, vol 72(6).

[865]  Chen KH, et al. Tangeretin suppresses IL-1beta-induced cyclooxygenase (COX)-2 expression through inhibition of p38 MAPK, JNK, and AKT activation in human lung carcinoma cells." Biochem Pharmacol. 2007, vol 73(2), pp 215-227.

[866]  Martinez CC, et al. "Treatment of metastatic melanoma B16F10 by the flavonoids tangeretin, rutin, and diosmin." J Agric Food Chem. 2005, vol 53(17), pp 6791-6797.

[867]  Ebrahimi A and Schluesener H. "Natural polyphenols against neurodegenerative disorders: Potentials and pitfalls." 2012, vol 11(2), pp 329-345.

[868]  Arafa el-SA, et al. "Tangeretin sensitizes cisplatin-resistant human ovarian cancer cells through downregulation of phosphoinositide 3-kinase/Akt signaling pathway." Cancer Res. 2009, vol 69(23), pp 8910-1917.

[869]  Datla KP, et al. "Tissue distribution and neuroprotective effects of citrus flavonoid tangeretin in a rat model of Parkinson's disease." Neuroreport. 2001, vol 12(17), pp 3871-3875.

[870]  Juhee Seo, et al. "Tangeretin, a citrus flavonoid, inhibits PGDF-BB-induced proliferation and migration of aortic smooth muscle cells by blocking AKT activation." European journal of Pharmacology. 2011, vol 673(1-3), pp 56-64.

[871]  Hirano T, et al. "Citrus flavone tangeretin inhibits leukaemic HL-60 cell growth partially through induction of apoptosis with less cytotoxicity on normal lymphocytes." Br J Cancer. 1995, vol 72(6).

[872]  Calomme M, et al. "Inhibition of Bacterial Mutagenesis by Citrus Flavonoids." Planta Med. 1996, vol 63(3), pp 222-226.

[873]  van Zanden JJ, et al. "Structural requirements for the flavonoid-mediated modulation of glutathione S-transferase P1-1 and GS-X pump activity in MCF7 breast cancer cells." Biochemical Pharmacology. 2004, vol 67(8), pp 1607-1617.

[874]  Kawaii S, et al. "Antiproliferative Activity of Flavonoids on Several Cancer Cell Lines." Bioscience, Biotechnolog, and Biochemistry. 1999, vol 63(5P), pp 896-899.

[875]  Yoshiaki Miyake, et al. "Lipid-Lowering Effect of Eriocitrin, the Main Flavonoid in Lemon Fruit, in Rats on a High-Fat and High-Cholesterol Diet." Journal of Food Science. 2006, vol 71(9), pp S633-S637.

[876]  Nakashima S, et al. "Melanogenesis inhibitors from the desert plant Anastatica hierochuntica in B16 melanoma cells." Bioorg Med Chem. 2010, vol 18(6), pp 1337-1345.

[877]  Williams HL, et al. "ERIODICTYOL GLYCOSIDE IN THE TREATMENT OF MENIERE'S DISEASE." Ann Otol Rhinol Laryngol. 1963, vol 72, pp 1082-1101.

Alan R. Gaby. "Integrative Approaches to Ménière's Disease." Integrative Medicine. 2009, vol 8(2), pp 30-32.

[878]  Sanchez de Rojas VR, et al. "Isolation of Vasodilatory Active Flavonoids from the Traditional Remedy Satureja obovata." Planta Med. 1996, vol 62(3), pp 272-274.

[879]  Alan R Gaby. "Integrative Approaches to Ménière's Disease." Integrative Medicine. 2009, vol 8(2), pp 30-32.

[880]  van Baren C, et al. "Triterpenic Acids and Flavonoids from *Satureja parvifolia*. Evaluation of their Antiprotozoal Activity." Naturforsch. 2006, vol 61c, pp 189-192.

[881]  Lee ER, et al. Cytoprotective effect of eriodictyol in UV-irradiated keratinocytes via phosphatase-dependent modulation of both the p38 MAPK and Akt signaling pathways. Cell Physiol Biochem. 2011, vol 27(5), pp 513-524.

[882]  Kawaii S, et al. "Antiproliferative Activity of Flavonoids on Several Cancer Cell Lines." Bioscience, Biotechnology, and Biochemistry. 1999, vol 63(5), pp 896-699.

[883]  Garg A, et al. "Chemistry and pharmacology of the citrus bioflavonoid hesperidin." Phytotherapy Research. 2001, vol 15(8), pp 655-669.

[884]  Garg A, et al. "Chemistry and pharmacology of the citrus bioflavonoid hesperidin." Phytotherapy Research. 2001, vol 15(8), pp 655-669.

885   Ravichandran G, et al. " Evaluation of the efficacy and safety of "Anti-Wrinkle cream" in the treatment of facial skin wrinkles: A prospective, open, phase III clinical trial." <u>The Antiseptic.</u> 2005, vol 102(2), pp 65-70.

886   Choong Jae Lee et al. Hesperidin suppressed proliferations of both Human breast cancer and androgen-dependent prostate cancer cells  Phytotherapy Research. 2010, vol 24 (S1), pp S15-S19.

887   Dimpfel W. "Hesperidin for prophylaxis and treatment of diseases of the central nervous system, in particular Alzheimer's and Parkinson's diseases, for therapy after stroke as well as for chronic pain." European Patent Application EP1621201. Date 7/28/2004.

888   M Mamani-Matsuda et al. Therapeutic and preventive properties of quercetin in experimental arthritis correlate with decreased macrophage inflammatory mediators. 2006, vol 72 (10), pp 1304-1310.

889   Uehara M. "Prevention of osteoporosis by foods and dietary supplements. Hesperidin and bone metabolism." <u>Clin Calcium</u>. 2006, vol 16(10), pp 1669-1676.

890   Choong Jae Lee et al. Hesperidin suppressed proliferations of both Human breast cancer and androgen-dependent prostate cancer cells  Phytotherapy Research. 2010, vol 24 (S1), pp S15-S19.

891   none


892   Masaki Yamamoto, et al. "Glucosyl hesperidin prevents endothelial dysfunction and oxidative stress in spontaneously hypertensive rats." <u>Nutrition.</u> 2008, vol 24(5), pp 470-476.

893   Dimpfel W. "Hesperidin for prophylaxis and treatment of diseases of the central nervous system, in particular Alzheimer's and Parkinson's diseases, for therapy after stroke as well as for chronic pain." European Patent Application EP1621201. Date 7/28/2004.

894   Kiichiro Kawaguchi, et al. "Suppression of Collagen-Induced Arthritis by Oral Administration of the Citrus Flavonoid Hesperidin." <u>Planta Med.</u> 2006, vol 72(5), pp 477-489.

895   Park HJ, et al. " Apoptotic effect of hesperidin through caspase3 activation in human colon cancer cells, SNU-C4." <u>Phytomedicine.</u> 2008, vol 15(1-2), pp 147-151.

896   Akiyama S, et al. Hypoglycemic and hypolipidemic effects of hesperidin and cyclodextrin-clathrated hesperetin in Goto-Kakizaki rats with type 2 diabetes. Biosci Biotechnol Biochem. 2009, vol 73(12), pp 2779-2782.

897   Masaki Yamamoto, et al. "Glucosyl hesperidin prevents endothelial dysfunction and oxidative stress in spontaneously hypertensive rats." <u>Nutrition.</u> 2008, vol 24(5), pp 470-476.

898   Xiaoyan Wang, et al. "Anti-influenza agents from plants and traditional Chinese medicine." <u>Phytotherapy Research.</u> 2006, vol 20(5), pp 335-341.

899   Sharma A, et al. "Drug discovery against H1N1 virus (influenza A virus) via computational virtual screening approach." <u>Medicinal Chemistry Research.</u> 2011, vol 20(9), pp 1445-1449.

900   Garg A, et al. "Chemistry and pharmacology of the citrus bioflavonoid hesperidin." <u>Phytotherapy Research.</u> 2001, vol 15(8), pp 655-669.

901   Kamaraj S et al. Antioxidant and anticancer efficacy of hesperidin in benzo(a)pyrene induced lung carcinogenesis in mice. Investigational New Drugs. 2009, vol 27 (3), pp 214-222.

902   Garg A, et al. "Chemistry and pharmacology of the citrus bioflavonoid hesperidin." <u>Phytotherapy Research.</u> 2001, vol 15(8), pp 655-669.

903   Simka M. "Blood Brain Barrier Compromise with Endothelial Inflammation may Lead to Autoimmune Loss of Myelin during Multiple Sclerosis." <u>Current Neurovascular Research.</u> 2009, vol 6(2), pp 132-139(8). http://www.ingentaconnect.com/content/ben/cnr/2009/00000006/00000002/art00008

904   Uehara M. "Prevention of osteoporosis by foods and dietary supplements. Hesperidin and bone metabolism." <u>Clin Calcium.</u> 2006, vol 16(10), pp 1669-1676.

[905]   Dimpfel W. "Hesperidin for prophylaxis and treatment of diseases of the central nervous system, in particular Alzheimer's and Parkinson's diseases, for therapy after stroke as well as for chronic pain." European Patent Application EP1621201. Date 7/28/2004.

[906]   Kiichiro Kawaguchi, et al. "Suppression of Collagen-Induced Arthritis by Oral Administration of the Citrus Flavonoid Hesperidin." Planta Med. 2006, vol 72(5), pp 477-489.

[907]   Shapiro H MD et al. "Polyphenols in the prevention and treatment of sepsis syndromes: Rationale and pre-clinical evidence." Nutrition. 2009, vol 25 (11), pp 981-997.

[908]   Garg A, et al. "Chemistry and pharmacology of the citrus bioflavonoid hesperidin." Phytotherapy Research. 2001, vol 15(8), pp 655-669.

[909]   Dimpfel W. "Hesperidin for prophylaxis and treatment of diseases of the central nervous system, in particular Alzheimer's and Parkinson's diseases, for therapy after stroke as well as for chronic pain." European Patent Application EP1621201. Date 7/28/2004.

[910]   Ravichandran G, et al. " Evaluation of the efficacy and safety of "Anti-Wrinkle cream" in the treatment of facial skin wrinkles: A prospective, open, phase III clinical trial." The Antiseptic. 2005, vol 102(2), pp 65-70.

[911]   Horcajada MN, et al. "Hesperidin inhibits ovariectomized-induced osteopenia and shows differential effects on bone mass and strength in young and adult intact rats." J Appl Physiol. 2008, vol 104(3), pp 648-654.

[912]   Koyuncu H et al. "Preventive effect of hesperidin against inflammation in CD-1 mouse skin caused by tumor promoter." Anticancer Research. 1999, vol 19 (4B), pp 3237-3241.

[913]   Ravichandran G, et al. " Evaluation of the efficacy and safety of "Anti-Wrinkle cream" in the treatment of facial skin wrinkles: A prospective, open, phase III clinical trial." The Antiseptic. 2005, vol 102(2), pp 65-70.

[914]   Heo HJ, et al. "Naringenin from *Citrus junos* Has an Inhibitory Effect on Acetylcholinesterase and a Mitigating Effect on Amnesia." Dement Geriatr Cogn Disord. 2004, vol 17, pp 151-157.

[915]  Heo HJ, et al. "Naringenin from *Citrus junos* Has an Inhibitory Effect on Acetylcholinesterase and a Mitigating Effect on Amnesia." <u>Dement Geriatr Cogn Disord.</u> 2004, vol 17, pp 151-157.

[916]  Anderson W, et al. "Investigation of the Anxiolytic Effects of Naringenin, a Component of Mentha Aquatica, in the Male Sprague-Dawley Rat." <u>Holistic Nursing Practice.</u> 2012, vol 26(1), pp 52-57.

[917]  Mulvihill EE, et al. "Naringenin Decreases Progression of Atherosclerosis by Improving Dyslipidemia in High-Fat–Fed Low-Density Lipoprotein Receptor–Null Mice." <u>Arteriosclerosis, Thrombosis, and Vascular Biology.</u> 2010, vol 30, pp 742-748.

[918]  Harmon AW and Patel YM. "Naringenin Inhibits Glucose Uptake in MCF-7 Breast Cancer Cells: A Mechanism for Impaired Cellular Proliferation." <u>Breast Cancer Research and Treatment.</u> 2004, vol 85(2), pp 103-110.

[919]  Chul-Ho Lee, et al. "Anti-Atherogenic Effect of Citrus Flavonoids, Naringin and Naringenin, Associated with Hepatic ACAT and Aortic VCAM-1 and MCP-1 in High Cholesterol-Fed Rabbits." <u>Biochemical and Biophysical Research Communications.</u> 2001, vol 284(3), pp 681-688.

[920]  Wang W, et al. "Individual and Interactive Effects of Apigenin Analogs on G2/M Cell-Cycle Arrest in Human Colon Carcinoma Cell Lines." <u>Nutrition and Cancer.</u> 2004, vol 48(1), pp 106-114.

[921]  Chul-Ho Lee, et al. "Anti-Atherogenic Effect of Citrus Flavonoids, Naringin and Naringenin, Associated with Hepatic ACAT and Aortic VCAM-1 and MCP-1 in High Cholesterol-Fed Rabbits." <u>Biochemical and Biophysical Research Communications.</u> 2001, vol 284(3), pp 681-688.

[922]  Ii-Tao Yi, et al. "Involvement of monoaminergic system in the antidepressant-like effect of the flavonoid naringenin in mice." <u>Progress in Neuro-Psychopharmacology and Biological Psychiatry.</u> 2010, vol 34(7), pp 1223-1228.

923   Ortiz-Andrade RR, et al. "Antidiabetic and toxicological evaluations of naringenin in normoglycaemic and NIDDM rat models and its implications on extra-pancreatic glucose regulation." <u>Diabetes, obesity and Metabolism.</u> 2008, vol 10(11), pp 1097-1104.

924   Jayaraman J, et al. "Potential beneficial effect of naringenin on lipid peroxidation and antioxidant status in rats with ethanol-induced hepatotoxicity." <u>Journal of Pharmacy and Pharmacology.</u> 2009, vol 61(10), pp 1383-1390.

925   Duthie GG, et al. " Plant polyphenols in cancer and heart disease: implications as nutritional antioxidants." <u>Nutrition Research Reviews.</u> 2000, vol 13, pp 79-106.

926   Goldwasser J, et al. "Naringenin inhibits the assembly and long-term production of infectious hepatitis C virus particles through a PPAR-mediated mechanism." <u>J Hepatol</u>. 2011, vol 55 (5), pp 963-971.

927   Nobuyuki Yamagishi, et al. "Naringenin Inhibits the Aggregation of Expanded Polyglutamine Tract-Containing Protein through the Induction of Endoplasmic Reticulum Chaperone GRP78." <u>Biological and Pharmaceutical Bulletin.</u> 2012, vol 35(10), pp 1836-1830.

928   Mulvihill EE, et al. "Naringenin Prevents Dyslipidemia, Apolipoprotein B Overproduction, and Hyperinsulinemia in LDL Receptor–Null Mice With Diet-Induced Insulin Resistance." <u>Diabetes.</u> 2009, vol 58(10), pp 2198-2210.

929   Gangjun Du, et al. "Naringenin: A Potential Immunomodulator for Inhibiting Lung Fibrosis and Metastasis." <u>Cancer Research.</u> 2009, vol 69, p 3205.

930   Cheng-Yun Jin, et al. "Naringenin up-regulates the expression of death receptor 5 and enhances TRAIL-induced apoptosis in human lung cancer A549 cells. " <u>Molecular Nutrition & Food Research.</u> 2011, vol 55(2), pp 300-309.

931   Mulvihill EE, et al. "Naringenin Prevents Dyslipidemia, Apolipoprotein B Overproduction, and Hyperinsulinemia in LDL Receptor–Null Mice With Diet-Induced Insulin Resistance." <u>Diabetes.</u> 2009, vol 58(10), pp 2198-2210.

932   Zbarsky V, et al. "Neuroprotective properties of the natural phenolic antioxidants curcumin and naringenin but not quercetin and fisetin in a 6-OHDA model of Parkinson's disease." <u>Free Radical Research.</u> 2005, vol 39(10), pp 1119-1125.

933   Kun Gao, et al. "The citrus flavonoid naringenin stimulates DNA repair in prostate cancer cells." Journal of Nutritional Biochemistry. 2006, vol 17(2), pp 89-95.

934   Kun Gao, et al. "The citrus flavonoid naringenin stimulates DNA repair in prostate cancer cells." Journal of Nutritional Biochemistry. 2006, vol 17(2), pp 89-95.

935   Chul-Ho Lee, et al. "Anti-Atherogenic Effect of Citrus Flavonoids, Naringin and Naringenin, Associated with Hepatic ACAT and Aortic VCAM-1 and MCP-1 in High Cholesterol-Fed Rabbits." <u>Biochemical and Biophysical Research Communications</u>. 2001, vol 284(3), pp 681-688.

936   Li-Tao Yi, et al. "Involvement of monoaminergic system in the antidepressant-like effect of the flavonoid naringenin in mice." <u>Progress in Neuro-Psychopharmacology and Biological Psychiatry.</u> 2010, vol 34(7), pp 1223-1228.

937   Fa Yun Zhang, et al. "Naringenin Enhances the Anti-Tumor Effect of Doxorubicin Through Selectively Inhibiting the Activity of Multidrug Resistance-Associated Proteins but not P-glycoprotein." <u>Pharmaceutical Research.</u> 2009, vol 26(4), pp 914-925.

938   Duarte N, et al. "Phenolic compounds as selective antineoplasic agents against multidrug-resistant human cancer cells." <u>Planta Med.</u> 2010, vol 76(10), pp 975-980.

939   Anderson W, et al. "Investigation of the Anxiolytic Effects of Naringenin, a Component of Mentha Aquatica, in the Male Sprague-Dawley Rat." <u>Holistic Nursing Practice.</u> 2012, vol 26(1), pp 52-57.

940   Zbarsky V, et al. "Neuroprotective properties of the natural phenolic antioxidants curcumin and naringenin but not quercetin and fisetin in a 6-OHDA model of Parkinson's disease." <u>Free Radical Research.</u> 2005, vol 39(10), pp 1119-1125.

[941]  Harmon AW and Patel YM. "Naringenin Inhibits Glucose Uptake in MCF-7 Breast Cancer Cells: A Mechanism for Impaired Cellular Proliferation." Breast Cancer Research and Treatment. 2004, vol 85(2), pp 103-110.

[942]  Kren V and Walterova D. "Silybin and Solitarian - New Effects and Applications." Biomedical Papers. 2005, vol 149 (1), pp 29-41.

[943]  Pesakhov S, et al. "Distinct combinatorial effects of the plant polyphenols curcumin, carnosic acid, and silibinin on proliferation and apoptosis in acute myeloid leukemia cells." Nutr Cancer.  2010, vol 62(6), pp 811-824.

[944]  Kren V and Walterova D. "Silybin and Solitarian - New Effects and Applications." Biomedical Papers. 2005, vol 149 (1), pp 29-41.

[945]  Yin F, et al.  "Silibinin: a novel inhibitor of AB Aggregation."  Neurochem Int. 2011, vol 58(3), pp 399-403.

[946]  Wellington K and Jarvis B. "Silymarin: A Review of its Clinical Properties in the Management of Hepatic Disorders." DioDrugs. 2001, vol 15(7), pp 465-489.

[947]  Lu P, et al. "Silibinin prevents amyloid $\beta$ peptide-induced memory impairment and oxidative stress in mice." British Journal of Pharmacology. 2009, vol 157(7), pp 1270-1277.

[948]  Flaig TW, et al. "A phase I and pharmacokinetic study of silybin-phytosome in prostate cancer patients." Investigational New Drugs. 2007, vol 25(2), pp 139-146.

[949]  Cooray HC, et al. "Interaction of the breast cancer resistance protein with plant polyphenols." Biochemical and Biophysical Research Communications. 2004, vol 317(1), pp 269-275.

[950]  Kren V and Walterova D. "Silybin and Solitarian - New Effects and Applications." Biomedical Papers. 2005, vol 149 (1), pp 29-41.

[951]  Ibid.

[952]  Schrieber SJ, et al. "Differences in the Disposition of Silymarin Between Patients with Non-Alcoholic Fatty Liver Disease and Chronic Hepatitis C." DMD. 2011. Dmd.111.040212.

953   Carmela Loguercio and Davide Festi. "Silybin and the liver: From basic research to clinical practice." <u>World J Gastroenterol.</u> 2011, vol 17(18), pp 2288-2301.

954   Flaig TW, et al. "A phase I and pharmacokinetic study of silybin-phytosome in prostate cancer patients." <u>Investigational New Drugs.</u> 2007, vol 25(2), pp 139-146.

955   Kren V and Walterova D. "Silybin and Solitarian - New Effects and Applications." <u>Biomedical Papers.</u> 2005, vol 149 (1), pp 29-41.

956   Wen-Jun Duan, et al. "Silibinin activated ROS-p38-NF-KB positive feedback and induced autophagic death in human fibro sarcoma HT1080 cells." <u>Journal of Asian Natural Products Research.</u> 2011, vol 13(1).

957   Kren V and Walterova D. "Silybin and Solitarian - New Effects and Applications." <u>Biomedical Papers.</u> 2005, vol 149 (1), pp 29-41.

958   Ibid.

959   Ramakrishnan G, et al. "Silymarin inhibited proliferation and induced apoptosis in hepatic cancer cells." <u>Cell Prolif</u>. 209, vol 42(2), pp 229-240.

960   Wellington K and Jarvis B. "Silymarin: A Review of its Clinical Properties in the Management of Hepatic Disorders." <u>DioDrugs.</u> 2001, vol 15(7), pp 465-489.

961   Kren V and Walterova D. "Silybin and Solitarian - New Effects and Applications." <u>Biomedical Papers.</u> 2005, vol 149 (1), pp 29-41.

962   Ibid.

963   Schrieber SJ, et al. "Differences in the Disposition of Silymarin Between Patients with Non-Alcoholic Fatty Liver Disease and Chronic Hepatitis C." <u>DMD</u>. 2011. Dmd.111.040212.

964   Gallo D, et al. "Antitumour activity of the silybin-phosphatidylcholine complex, IdB 1016, against human ovarian cancer." <u>European Journal of Cancer.</u> 2003, vol 39(16), pp 2403-2410.

965   Kren V and Walterova D. "Silybin and Solitarian - New Effects and Applications." <u>Biomedical Papers.</u> 2005, vol 149 (1), pp 29-41.

966   Ibid.

967   Flaig TW, et al. "A phase I and pharmacokinetic study of silybin-hydrosome in prostate cancer patients." <u>Investigational New Drugs.</u> 2007, vol 25(2), pp 139-146.

968   Ibid.

969   Kren V and Walterova D. "Silybin and Solitarian - New Effects and Applications." <u>Biomedical Papers.</u> 2005, vol 149 (1), pp 29-41.

970   Ibid.

971   Ibid.

972   Ibid.

973   Ibid.

974   Kren V and Walterova D. "Silybin and Solitarian - New Effects and Applications." <u>Biomedical Papers.</u> 2005, vol 149 (1), pp 29-41.

975   Kren V and Walterova D. "Silybin and silymarin - new effects and applications." <u>Biomed Pap Med Fac Univ Palacky Olomouc Czech Repub</u>. 2005, vol 149(1), pp 29-41.

976   Kren V and Walterova D. "Silybin and Solitarian - New Effects and Applications." <u>Biomedical Papers.</u> 2005, vol 149 (1), pp 29-41.

977   Ibid.

978   Carmela Loguercio and Davide Festi. "Silybin and the liver: From basic research to clinical practice." <u>World J Gastroenterol.</u> 2011, vol 17(18), pp 2288-2301.

979   Ibid.

[980] Giridharan VV, et al. "Prevention of scopolamine-induced memory deficits by schisandrin B, an antioxidant lignan from Schisandra chinensis in mice." <u>Free Radical Research.</u> 2011, vol 45(8), pp 950-958.

[981] Touillaud MS, et al. "Dietary Lignan Intake and Postmenopausal Breast Cancer Risk by Estrogen and Progesterone Receptor Status." <u>Oxford Journals. JNCI J Natl Cancer Inst.</u> 2007, vol 99(6), pp 475-486.

[982] Peterson J, et al. "Dietary lignans: physiology and potential for cardiovascular disease risk reduction." <u>Nutrition Reviews.</u> 2010, vol 68(10), pp 571-603.

[983] Hongyan Qu, et al. "Lignans Are Involved in the Antitumor Activity of Wheat Bran in Colon Cancer SW480 Cells." <u>J Nutr.</u> 2005, vol 135(3), pp 598-602.

[984] Hongyan Qu, et al. "Lignans Are Involved in the Antitumor Activity of Wheat Bran in Colon Cancer SW480 Cells." <u>J Nutr.</u> 2005, vol 135(3), pp 598-602.

[985] Clifton P. "Cereal grains and legumes in the prevention of coronary heart disease and stroke: a review of the literature." <u>European Journal of Clinical Nutrition.</u> 2006, vol 60, pp 1145-1159.

[986] Montonen J, et al. "Whole-grain and fiber intake and the incidence of type 2 diabetes." <u>Am J Clin Nutr.</u> 2003, vol 77(3), pp 622-629.

[987] Alhassane Toure' and Xu Xueming. "Flaxseed Lignans: Source, Biosynthesis, Metabolism, Antioxidant Activity, Bio-Active Components, and Health Benefits." <u>Comprehensive Reviews in Food Science and Food Safety.</u> 2010, vol 9(3), pp 261-269.

[988] Clifton P. "Cereal grains and legumes in the prevention of coronary heart disease and stroke: a review of the literature." <u>European Journal of Clinical Nutrition.</u> 2006, vol 60, pp 1145-1159.

[989] Lee JC, et al. "Dietary flaxseed enhances antioxidant defenses and is protective in a mouse model of lung ischemia-reperfusion injury." <u>AJP - Lung Physiol.</u> 2007, vol 294(2), pp L255-L265.

[990] Suthar AC, et al. "Pharmacological activities of Genistein, an isoflavone from soy (Glycine max): part II--anti-cholesterol activity, effects on osteoporosis & menopausal symptoms." <u>Indian J Exp Biol.</u> 2001, vol 39(6), pp 520-525.

[991]  Ibid.

[992]  McCann SE, et al. "Intakes of Selected Nutrients and Food Groups and Risk of Ovarian Cancer." <u>Nutrition and Cancer.</u> 2001, vol 39 (1), pp 19-28.

[993]  Bahram H. Arjmandi. "The Role of Phytoestrogens in the Prevention and Treatment of Osteoporosis in Ovarian Hormone Deficiency." <u>J Am Coll Nutr.</u> 2001, vol 20(5), pp 3985-4025.

[994]  Lin X, et al. "Effect of mammalian lignans on the growth of prostate cancer cell lines." <u>Anticancer Research.</u> 2001, vol 21(6A), pp 3995-3999.

[995]  Clifton P. "Cereal grains and legumes in the prevention of coronary heart disease and stroke: a review of the literature." <u>European Journal of Clinical Nutrition.</u> 2006, vol 60, pp 1145-1159.

[996]  Thompson LU, et al. "Dietary Flaxseed Alters Tumor Biological Markers in Postmenopausal Breast Cancer." <u>Clin Cancer Res.</u> 2005, vol 11, p 3828.

[997]  Ibid.

[998]  Milder IE, et al. "Lignan contents of Dutch plant foods: a database including lariciresinol, pinoresinol, secoisolariciresinol and matairesinol." <u>Br J Nutr.</u> 2005, vol 93(3), pp 393-402.

[999]  Ahotupa M, et al. "METHOD OF INHIBITING OVERACTIVITY OF PHAGOCYTES OR LYMPHOCTES IN AN INDIVIDUAL," US Patent 7,008,666 B2, 2006, filed in 2001.

[1000]  Ahotupa M, et al. "METHOD OF INHIBITING OVERACTIVITY OF PHAGOCYTES OR LYMPHOCTES IN AN INDIVIDUAL," US Patent 7,008,666 B2, 2006, filed in 2001.

[1001]  Thompson LU, et al. "Dietary Flaxseed Alters Tumor Biological Markers in Postmenopausal Breast Cancer." <u>Clinical Cancer Res.</u> 2005, vol 11, pp 3828.

[1002]  van der Schouw Y, et al. "Cardiovascular Disease in Women  Prospective Study on Usual Dietary Phytoestrogen Intake and Cardiovascular Disease Risk in Western Women." <u>Circulation.</u> 2005, vol 111, pp 465-471.

[1003]  Lechner D, et al. "Phytoestrogens and Colorectal Cancer Prevention." Vitamins & Hormones. 2005, vol 79, pp 169-198.

[1004]  van der Schouw Y, et al. "Cardiovascular Disease in Women  Prospective Study on Usual Dietary Phytoestrogen Intake and Cardiovascular Disease Risk in Western Women." Circulation. 2005, vol 111, pp 465-471.

[1005]  Shin-Ichi Katsuda, et al. "Chemopreventive Effects of Hydroxymatairesinol on Uterine Carcinogenesis in Donryu Rats." Exp Biol Med. 2004, vol 229(5), pp 417-424.

[1006]  Ahotupa M, et al. "METHOD OF INHIBITING OVERACTIVITY OF PHAGOCYTES OR LYMPHOCTES IN AN INDIVIDUAL," US Patent 7,008,666 B2, 2006, filed in 2001.

[1007]  Bylund A, et al. "Anticancer Effects of a Plant Lignan 7-Hydroxymatairesinol on a Prostate Cancer Model *In Vivo*." Exp Biol Med. 2005(3), pp 217-223.

[1008]  Saarinen NM, et al. "Hydroxymatairesinol, a Novel Enterolactone Precursor With Antitumor Properties From Coniferous Tree (Picea abies)." Nutrition and Cancer. 2000, vol 36920, PP 207-216.

[1009]  Ahotupa M, et al. "METHOD OF INHIBITING OVERACTIVITY OF PHAGOCYTES OR LYMPHOCTES IN AN INDIVIDUAL," US Patent 7,008,666 B2, 2006, filed in 2001.

[1010]  Kucukboyaci N, et al. "Assessment of Enzyme Inhibitory and Antioxidant Activities of Lignans from Taxus baccata L." Z. Naturforsch. 2010, vol 65c, pp 187-194.

[1011]  Saarinen NM, et al. "Dietary lariciresinol attenuates mammary tumor growth and reduces blood vessel density in human MCF-7 breast cancer xenografts and carcinogen-induced mammary tumors in rats." Int J Cancer. 2008, vol 123(5), pp 1196-1204.

[1012]  Bomi Hwang, et al. "Antifungal activity of lariciresinol derived from Sambucus williamsii and their membrane-active mechanisms in Candida albicans." Biochemical and Biophysical Research Communications. 2011, vol 410, vol 3, pp 489-493.

[1013]  Milder IEJ, et al. "Intake of the Plant Lignans Secoisolariciresinol, Matairesinol, Lariciresinol, and Pinoresinol in Dutch Men and Women." <u>JNutr.</u> 2006, vol 135(5), pp 1202-1205.

[1014]  Hausott B, et al. "Naturally occurring lignans efficiently induce apoptosis in colorectal tumor cells." <u>Journal of Cancer Research and Clinical Oncology.</u> 2003, vol 129(10), pp 569-576.

[1015]  Rui Hai Liu. "Whole grain phytochemicals and health." <u>Journal of Cereal Science.</u> 2007, vol 469(3), pp 207-219

[1016]  US Patent # US2008/0057140. Inventor Mikko Unkila. "Use of a Lignan for the manufacture of a compositon for preventing or alleviating of symptoms relating to estrogen deficiency." Pub date Mar. 6, 2008.

[1017]  Saarinen NM, et al. "Dietary lariciresinol attenuates mammary tumor growth and reduces blood vessel density in human MCF-7 breast cancer xenografts and carcinogen-induced mammary tumors in rats." <u>Int J Cancer.</u> 2008, vol 123(5), pp 1196-1204.

[1018]  Bandera EV, et al. "Phytoestrogen consumption from foods and supplements and epithelial ovarian cancer risk: a population-based case control study." <u>BMC Womens Health</u>. 2011, vol 11.40.

[1019]  Ki Hyun Kim, et al. "Biological evaluation of phenolic constituents from the trunk of *Berberis koreana*." <u>Bioorganic & Medicinal Chemistry Letters.</u> 2011, vol 21(8), pp 2270-2273.

[1020]  Hedelin M, et al. "Dietary Phytoestrogen, Serum Enterolactone and Risk of Prostate Cancer: The Cancer Prostate Sweden Study (Sweden)." <u>Cancer Causes & Control.</u> 2006, vol 17(2), pp 169-180.

[1021]  Gurbuz I, et al. "Anti-ulcerogenic Lignans from Taxus baccata L." <u>Z. Naturforsch.</u> 2004, vol 59c, pp 233-236.

[1022]  Saarinen NM, et al. "Dietary lariciresinol attenuates mammary tumor growth and reduces blood vessel density in human MCF-7 breast cancer xenografts and carcinogen-induced mammary tumors in rats." <u>Int J Cancer.</u> 2008, vol 123(5), pp 1196-1204.

[1023]   Gurbuz I, et al. "Anti-ulcerogenic Lignans from Taxus baccata L." <u>Z. Naturforsch.</u> 2004, vol 59c, pp 233-236.

[1024]   Ibid.

Kucukboyaci N, et al. "Assessment of Enzyme Inhibitory and Antioxidant Activities of Lignans from Taxus baccata L." <u>Z. Naturforsch.</u> 2010, vol 65c, pp 187-194.

[1025]   Ki Hyun Kim, et al. "Biological evaluation of phenolic constituents from the trunk of *Berberis koreana*." <u>Bioorganic & Medicinal Chemistry Letters.</u> 2011, vol 21(8), pp 2270-2273.

[1026]   Ahotupa M, et al. "METHOD OF INHIBITING OVERACTIVITY OF PHAGOCYTES OR LYMPHOCTES IN AN INDIVIDUAL," US Patent 7,008,666 B2, 2006, filed in 2001.

[1027]   Ibid..

[1028]   Ilja CW and Hollman PCH. "Polyphenols and disease risk in epidemiologic studies." <u>Am J Clin Nutr.</u> 2005, vol 81(1), pp 2175-2255.

[1029]   Mei J, et al. "High Dietary Phytoestrogen Intake Is Associated with Higher Bone Mineral Density in Postmenopausal but Not Premenopausal Women." <u>JCEM.</u> 2001, vol 8(11), pp 5217-5221.

[1030]   McCann SE, et al. "Dietary intakes of total and specific lignans are associated with clinical breast tumor characteristics." <u>J Nutr.</u> 2012, vol 142(1), pp 91-98.

[1031]   Milder IE, et al. "Intakes of 4 dietary lignans and cause-specific and all-cause mortality in the Zutphen Elderly Study." <u>Am J Clin Nutr.</u> 2006, vol 84(2), pp 400-405.

[1032]   Ibid.

[1033]   Saleh F, et al. "Phytoestrogen intake and cardiovascular risk markers in Bangladeshi postmenopausal women." <u>Mymensingh Med J.</u> 2011, vol 20(2), pp 219-225.

[1034]   Ilja CW and Hollman PCH. "Polyphenols and disease risk in epidemiologic studies." <u>Am J Clin Nutr.</u> 2005, vol 81(1), pp 2175-2255.

1035   Milder IE, et al. "Intakes of 4 dietary lignans and cause-specific and all-cause mortality in the Zutphen Elderly Study." <u>Am J Clin Nutr.</u> 2006, vol 84(2), pp 400-405.

1036   Rui Hai Liu. "Whole grain phytochemicals and health." <u>Journal of Cereal Science.</u> 2007, vol 469(3), pp 207-219

1037   Ilja CW and Hollman PCH. "Polyphenols and disease risk in epidemiologic studies." <u>Am J Clin Nutr.</u> 2005, vol 81(1), pp 2175-2255.

1038   Knight DC and Eden JA. "A Review of the Clinical Effects of Phytoestrogens." <u>Obstetrics & Gynecology.</u> 1996, vol 87(5).

1039   McCann SE, et al. "Risk of Human Ovarian Cancer Is Related to Dietary Intake of Selected Nutrients, Phytochemicals and Food Groups." <u>J Nutr.</u> 2002, vol 122(6), pp 1927-1942.

1040   Ahotupa M, et al. "METHOD OF INHIBITING OVERACTIVITY OF PHAGOCYTES OR LYMPHOCTES IN AN INDIVIDUAL," US Patent 7,008,666 B2, 2006, filed in 2001.

1041   Magee PJ and Rowland IR. "Phyto-oestrogens, their mechanism of action: current evidence for a role in breast and prostate cancer." <u>British Journal of Nutrition.</u> 2004, vol 91(4), pp 513-531.

1042   Ilja CW and Hollman PCH. "Polyphenols and disease risk in epidemiologic studies." <u>Am J Clin Nutr.</u> 2005, vol 81(1), pp 2175-2255.

1043   Pellegrini N, et al. "Intake of the plant lignans matairesinol, secoisolariciresinol, pinoresinol, and lariciresinol in relation to vascular inflammation and endothelial dysfunction in middle age-elderly men and post-menopausal women living in Northern Italy." <u>Nutrition, metabolism and Cardiovascular Disease.</u> 2010, vol 20(1), pp 64-71.

1044   Hyo Won Jung, et al. "Pinoresinol from the fruits of *Forsythia koreana* inhibits inflammatory responses in LPS-activated microglia." <u>Neuroscience Letters.</u> 2010, vol 480(3), pp 215-220.

1045   Paska C, et al. "Pinoresinol from Ipomoea Cairica Cell Cultures." <u>Natural Product Letters.</u> 2002, vol 16, pp 359-363.

[1046]   Milder IEJ, et al. "Intake of the Plant Lignans Secoisolariciresinol, Matairesinol, Lariciresinol, and Pinoresinol in Dutch Men and Women." <u>JNutr.</u> 2006, vol 135(5), pp 1202-1205.

[1047]   Fini L, et al. "Chemopreventive properties of pinoresinol-rich olive oil involve a selective activation of the ATM-p53 cascade in colon cancer cell lines." <u>Carcinogenesis</u>. 2008, vol 29(1), pp 139-146.

[1048]   Rui Hai Liu. "Whole grain phytochemicals and health." <u>Journal of Cereal Science.</u> 2007, vol 469(3), pp 207-219

[1049]   US Patent # US2008/0057140. Inventor Mikko Unkila. "Use of a Lignan for the manufacture of a compositon for preventing or alleviating of symptoms relating to estrogen deficiency." Pub date Mar. 6, 2008.

[1050]   Sedlak E, et al. "Bioactive phenols in leaves of Forsythia species." <u>International Journal of Horticultural Science.</u> 2008, vol 14(3), pp 57-59.

[1051]   Greenway F, et al. "A clinical trial testing the safety and efficacy of a standardized Eucommia ulmoides Oliver bark extract to treat hypertension." <u>Altern Med Rev</u>. 2011, vol 16(4), pp 338-347.

[1052]   Hyo Won Jung, et al. "Pinoresinol from the fruits of *Forsythia koreana* inhibits inflammatory responses in LPS-activated microglia." <u>Neuroscience Letters</u>. 2010, vol 480(3), pp 215-220.

[1053]   Ibid.

[1054]   Hedelin M, et al. "Dietary Phytoestrogen, Serum Enterolactone and Risk of Prostate Cancer: The Cancer Prostate Sweden Study (Sweden)." <u>Cancer Causes & Control.</u> 2006, vol 17(2), pp 169-180.
http://link.springer.com/article/10.1007/s10552-005-0342-2#

[1055]   Hyo Won Jung, et al. "Pinoresinol from the fruits of *Forsythia koreana* inhibits inflammatory responses in LPS-activated microglia." <u>Neuroscience Letters</u>. 2010, vol 480(3), pp 215-220.

[1056]   Greenway F, et al. "A clinical trial testing the safety and efficacy of a standardized Eucommia ulmoides Oliver bark extract to treat hypertension." <u>Altern Med Rev</u>. 2011, vol 16(4), pp 338-347.

[1057]   Hyo Won Jung, et al. "Pinoresinol from the fruits of *Forsythia koreana* inhibits inflammatory responses in LPS-activated microglia." <u>Neuroscience Letters</u>. 2010, vol 480(3), pp 215-220.

[1058]   Janaswamy Madhusudana Rao, et al. US Patent.  US 6,489,514 B1, "(-)-Secoisolariciresinol as an antioxidant obtained from a new natural source namely STEREOSPERMUM PERSONATUM." Date Dec 3, 2002.

[1059]   Saikat Sen, et al. "Free Radicals, antioxidants, diseases and phytomedicines: current status and future prospect." <u>International Journal of Pharmaceutical Sciences Review and Research.</u> 2010, vol 3(1), pp 91-100.

[1060]   Prasad K. "Antioxidant activity of secoisolariciresinol diglucoside-derived metabolites, secoisolariciresinol, Enterodiol, and enterolactone." <u>International Journal of Angiology.</u>  2000, vol 9(4), pp 220-225.

[1061]   Zhang W, et al. "Effects of dietary flaxseed lignan extract on symptoms of benign prostatic hyperplasia." <u>J Med Food</u>. 2008, vol 11(2), pp 207-214.

[1062]   Chen J, et al. "Flaxseed and pure secoisolariciresinol diglucoside, but not flaxseed hull, reduce human breast tumor growth (MCF-7) in athymic mice." <u>J Nutr.</u> 2009, vol 139(11), pp 2061-2066.

[1063]   Janaswamy Madhusudana Rao, et al. US Patent.  US 6,489,514 B1, "(-)-Secoisolariciresinol as an antioxidant obtained from a new natural source namely STEREOSPERMUM PERSONATUM." Date Dec 3, 2002.

[1064]   YingJun Zhou, et al. "Vitexins, Nature-Derived Lignan Compounds, Induce Apoptosis and Suppress Tumor Growth." <u>Clinical Cancer Research.</u> 2009, vol 15, p 5161.

[1065]   Ayella A, et al. "Cytostatic inhibition of cancer cell growth by lignan secoisolariciresinol diglucoside." <u>Nutr Res</u>. 2010, vol 30(11), pp 762-769.

[1066]   Hongyan Qu, et al. "Lignans Are Involved in the Antitumor Activity of Wheat Bran in Colon Cancer SW480 Cells." <u>J Nutr.</u> 2005, vol 135(3), pp 598-602.

[1067]   Prasad K. "Reduction of Serum Cholesterol and Hypercholesterolemic Atherosclerosis in Rabbits by Secoisolariciresinol Diglucoside Isolated From Flaxseed." <u>Circulation.</u> 1999, vol 99, pp 1355-1362.

[1068]   Prasad K. "Antioxidant activity of secoisolariciresinol diglucoside-derived metabolites, secoisolariciresinol, Enterodiol, and enterolactone." <u>International Journal of Angiology.</u>  2000, vol 9(4), pp 220-225.

[1069]   Rui Hai Liu. "Whole grain phytochemicals and health." <u>Journal of Cereal Science.</u> 2007, vol 469(3), pp 207-219

[1070]   Eckart Eich. "Secondary Metabolites from Plants as Antiretroviral Agents: Promising Lead Structures for Anti-HIV Drugs of the Future." <u>Phytomedicines of Europe.</u> ACS Symposium Series. Chapter 8, 1998, pp 83-96.

[1071]   YingJun Zhou, et al. "Vitexins, Nature-Derived Lignan Compounds, Induce Apoptosis and Suppress Tumor Growth." <u>Clinical Cancer Research.</u> 2009, vol 15, p 5161.

[1072]   Fukumitsu S, et al. "Flaxseed lignan lowers blood cholesterol and decreases liver disease risk factors in moderately hypercholesterolemic men." <u>Nutr Res.</u> 2010, vol 30(7), pp 441-446.

[1073]   Prasad K. "Antioxidant activity of secoisolariciresinol diglucoside-derived metabolites, secoisolariciresinol, Enterodiol, and enterolactone." <u>International Journal of Angiology.</u>  2000, vol 9(4), pp 220-225.

[1074]   YingJun Zhou, et al. "Vitexins, Nature-Derived Lignan Compounds, Induce Apoptosis and Suppress Tumor Growth." <u>Clinical Cancer Research.</u> 2009, vol 15, p 5161.

[1075]   Fukumitsu S, et al. "Flaxseed lignan lowers blood cholesterol and decreases liver disease risk factors in moderately hypercholesterolemic men." <u>Nutrition Research.</u> 2010, vol 30(7), pp 441-446.

[1076]   Saikat Sen, et al. "Free Radicals, antioxidants, diseases and phytomedicines: current status and future prospect." <u>International Journal of Pharmaceutical Sciences Review and Research.</u> 2010, vol 3(1), pp 91-100.

1077  Riccio P, et al. "May Diet and Dietary Supplements Improve the Wellness of Multiple Sclerosis Patients? A Molecular Approach." <u>Autoimmune Diseases.</u> 2010, vol 2010, article ID 249842, 12 pages.

1078  YingJun Zhou, et al. "Vitexins, Nature-Derived Lignan Compounds, Induce Apoptosis and Suppress Tumor Growth." <u>Clinical Cancer Research.</u> 2009, vol 15, p 5161.

1079  Magee PJ and Rowland IR. "Phyto-oestrogens, their mechanism of action: current evidence for a role in breast and prostate cancer." <u>British Journal of Nutrition.</u> 2004, vol 91(4), pp 513-531.

1080  Janaswamy Madhusudana Rao, et al. US Patent.  US 6,489,514 B1, "(-)-Secoisolariciresinol as an antioxidant obtained from a new natural source namely STEREOSPERMUM PERSONATUM." Date Dec 3, 2002.

1081  Banskota AH, et al. "Secoisolariciresinol and isotaxiresinol inhibit tumor necrosis factor-a-dependent hepatic apoptosis in mice." <u>Life Sciences.</u> 2004, vol 74(22), pp 2781-2792.

1082  Fukumitsu S, et al. "Flaxseed lignan lowers blood cholesterol and decreases liver disease risk factors in moderately hypercholesterolemic men." <u>Nutrition Research.</u> 2010, vol 30(7), pp 441-446.

1083  Hongyan Qu, et al. "Lignans Are Involved in the Antitumor Activity of Wheat Bran in Colon Cancer SW480 Cells." <u>J Nutr.</u> 2005, vol 135(3), pp 598-602.

1084  Ibid.

1085  Janaswamy Madhusudana Rao, et al. US Patent.  US 6,489,514 B1, "(-)-Secoisolariciresinol as an antioxidant obtained from a new natural source namely STEREOSPERMUM PERSONATUM." Date Dec 3, 2002.

1086  Yamashita K, et al. "Sesamin and \alpha-tocopherol synergistically suppress lipid-peroxide in rats fed a high docosahexaenoic acid diet." <u>Life Science, Biochemistry and Biophysics, Biotechnology and Microbiology and Virology.</u> 2000, vol 11, Numbers 1-2-2000, pp 11-13.

[1087]   Matsumura Y, et al. "Antihypertensive effect of sesamin. III. Protection against development and maintenance of hypertension in stroke-prone spontaneously hypertensive rats." <u>Biological & Pharmaceutical Bulletin.</u> 1998, vol 21(5), pp 469-473.

[1088]   Harikumar KB, et al. "Sesamin Manifests Chemopreventive Effects through the Suppression of NF-κB–Regulated Cell Survival, Proliferation, Invasion, and Angiogenic Gene Products." <u>Molecular Cancer Research.</u> 2010, vol 8, p 751.

[1089]   Noguchi T, et al. "Effects of vitamin E and sesamin on hypertension and cerebral thrombogenesis in stroke-prone spontaneously hypertensive rats." <u>Hypertension Research: Official Journal of the Japanese Society of Hypertension.</u> 2001, vol 24(6), pp 735-742.

[1090]   Harikumar KB, et al. "Sesamin Manifests Chemopreventive Effects through the Suppression of NF-κB–Regulated Cell Survival, Proliferation, Invasion, and Angiogenic Gene Products." <u>Molecular Cancer Research.</u> 2010, vol 8, p 751.

[1091]   Ibid.

[1092]   Prachya Kongtawelert. "PHYTOCHEMICAL COMPOSITIONS INCLUDING SESAMIN FOR ANTI¬ INFLAMMATORY, ANTI-CYTOKINE STORM, AND OTHER USES." International Application No. PCT/SG2009/000340.  Filing Date: 14.09.2009. Publication Date: 17.03.2011.  Pub. No: WO/2011/031237.

[1093]   Harikumar KB, et al. "Sesamin Manifests Chemopreventive Effects through the Suppression of NF-κB–Regulated Cell Survival, Proliferation, Invasion, and Angiogenic Gene Products." <u>Molecular Cancer Research.</u> 2010, vol 8, p 751.

[1094]   Prachya Kongtawelert. "PHYTOCHEMICAL COMPOSITIONS INCLUDING SESAMIN FOR ANTI¬ INFLAMMATORY, ANTI-CYTOKINE STORM, AND OTHER USES." US Pantent 2012/0178712 A1. Pub Date: Jul. 12, 2012.

[1095]   Ibid.

[1096]   Harikumar KB, et al. "Sesamin Manifests Chemopreventive Effects through the Suppression of NF-κB–Regulated Cell Survival, Proliferation, Invasion, and Angiogenic Gene Products." <u>Molecular Cancer Research.</u> 2010, vol 8, p 751.

[1097]  Akimoto K, et al. "Protective Effects of Sesamin against Liver Damage Caused by Alcohol or Carbon Tetrachloride in Rodents." <u>Nutrition & Metabolism</u>. 1993, vol 37(4), pp 218-224.

[1098]  Hirose N, et al. "Inhibition of cholesterol absorption and synthesis in rats by sesamin." <u>The Journal of Lipid Research.</u> 1999, vol 32, pp 629-638.

[1099]  Harikumar KB, et al. "Sesamin Manifests Chemopreventive Effects through the Suppression of NF-κB–Regulated Cell Survival, Proliferation, Invasion, and Angiogenic Gene Products." <u>Molecular Cancer Research.</u> 2010, vol 8, p 751.

[1100]  Ibid.

[1101]  Lahaie-collins V, et al. "Sesamin Modulates Tyrosine Hydroxylase, Superoxide Dismutase, Catalase, Inducible No Synthase and Interleukin-6 Expression in Dopaminergic Cells Under Mpp$^+$-Induced Oxidative Stress." <u>Oxidative Medicine and Cellular Lonevity.</u> 2008, vol 1(1), pp 54-62.

[1102]  Harikumar KB, et al. "Sesamin Manifests Chemopreventive Effects through the Suppression of NF-κB–Regulated Cell Survival, Proliferation, Invasion, and Angiogenic Gene Products." <u>Molecular Cancer Research.</u> 2010, vol 8, p 751.

[1103]  Lahaie-collins V, et al. "Sesamin Modulates Tyrosine Hydroxylase, Superoxide Dismutase, Catalase, Inducible No Synthase and Interleukin-6 Expression in Dopaminergic Cells Under Mpp$^+$-Induced Oxidative Stress." <u>Oxidative Medicine and Cellular Lonevity.</u> 2008, vol 1(1), pp 54-62.

[1104]  Harikumar KB, et al. "Sesamin Manifests Chemopreventive Effects through the Suppression of NF-κB–Regulated Cell Survival, Proliferation, Invasion, and Angiogenic Gene Products." <u>Molecular Cancer Research.</u> 2010, vol 8, p 751.

[1105]  Matsumura Y, et al. "Antihypertensive effect of sesamin. III. Protection against development and maintenance of hypertension in stroke-prone spontaneously hypertensive rats." <u>Biological & Pharmaceutical Bulletin.</u> 1998, vol 21(5), pp 469-473.

[1106]  Matsumura Y, et al. "Antihypertensive effect of sesamin. III. Protection against development and maintenance of hypertension in stroke-prone spontaneously hypertensive rats." <u>Biological & Pharmaceutical Bulletin.</u> 1998, vol 21(5), pp 469-473.

1107   Noguchi T, et al. "Effects of vitamin E and sesamin on hypertension and cerebral thrombogenesis in stroke-prone spontaneously hypertensive rats." <u>Hypertension Research: Official Journal of the Japanese Society of Hypertension.</u> 2001, vol 24(6), pp 735-742.

1108   Ide T, et al. "Sesamin, a sesame lignan, decreases fatty acid synthesis in rat liver accompanying the down-regulation of sterol regulatory element binding protein-1.." <u>Biochimica et Biophysica Acta.</u> 2001, vol 1534(1), pp 1-13.

1109   Yamashita K, et al. "Sesamin and \alpha-tocopherol synergistically suppress lipid-peroxide in rats fed a high docosahexaenoic acid diet." <u>Life Science, Biochemistry and Biophysics, Biotechnology and Microbiology and Virology.</u> 2000, vol 11, Numbers 1-2-2000, pp 11-13.

1110   Prachya Kongtawelert. "PHYTOCHEMICAL COMPOSITIONS INCLUDING SESAMIN FOR ANTI¬ INFLAMMATORY, ANTI-CYTOKINE STORM, AND OTHER USES." International Application No. PCT/SG2009/000340.  Filing Date: 14.09.2009. Publication Date: 17.03.2011.  Pub. No: WO/2011/031237.

1111   Ibid.

1112   Matsumura Y, et al. "Antihypertensive effect of sesamin. III. Protection against development and maintenance of hypertension in stroke-prone spontaneously hypertensive rats." <u>Biological & Pharmaceutical Bulletin.</u> 1998, vol 21(5), pp 469-473.

1113   Harikumar KB, et al. "Sesamin Manifests Chemopreventive Effects through the Suppression of NF-κB–Regulated Cell Survival, Proliferation, Invasion, and Angiogenic Gene Products." <u>Molecular Cancer Research.</u> 2010, vol 8, p 751.

1114   Prachya Kongtawelert. "PHYTOCHEMICAL COMPOSITIONS INCLUDING SESAMIN FOR ANTI¬ INFLAMMATORY, ANTI-CYTOKINE STORM, AND OTHER USES." International Application No. PCT/SG2009/000340.  Filing Date: 14.09.2009. Publication Date: 17.03.2011.  Pub. No: WO/2011/031237.

1115   Harikumar KB, et al. "Sesamin Manifests Chemopreventive Effects through the Suppression of NF-κB–Regulated Cell Survival, Proliferation, Invasion, and Angiogenic Gene Products." <u>Molecular Cancer Research.</u> 2010, vol 8, p 751.

1116   Lahaie-collins V, et al. "Sesamin Modulates Tyrosine Hydroxylase, Superoxide Dismutase, Catalase, Inducible No Synthase and Interleukin-6 Expression in Dopaminergic Cells Under Mpp$^+$-Induced Oxidative Stress." <u>Oxidative Medicine and Cellular Lonevity.</u> 2008, vol 1(1), pp 54-62.

1117   Zhou H, et al. "Serum carotenoids and risk of age-related macular degeneration in a chinese population sample." <u>Invest Ophthalmol.</u> 2011, vol 52(7), pp 4338-4344.

1118   Polidori MC, et al. "[Influence of vascular comorbidities on the antioxidant defense system in Alzheimer's disease]." <u>Dtsch Med Wochenschr.</u> 2012, vol 137(7), pp 305-308.

1119   Misso NLA, et al. "Plasma concentrations of dietary and nondietary antioxidants are low in severe asthma." <u>ERJ.</u> 2005, vol 26(2), pp 257-264.

1120   D'Odorico A, et al. "High plasma levels of α- and β-carotene are associated with a lower risk of atherosclerosis: Results from the Bruneck study." <u>Atherosclerosis.</u> 2000, vol 153(1), pp 231-2239.

1121   Larsson SC, et al. "Dietary carotenoids and risk of hormone receptor-defined breast cancer in a prospective cohort of Swedish women." <u>Eur J Cancer.</u> 2010, vol 46(6), pp 1079-1085.

1122   Tsiligianni IG and van der Molen T. "A systematic review of the role of vitamin insufficiencies and supplementation in COPD." <u>Respir Res.</u> 2010, 11:171.

1123   Narisawa T, et al."Inhibitory effects of natural carotenoids, α-carotene, β-carotene, lycopene and lutein, on colonic aberrant crypt foci formation in rats." <u>Cancer Letters.</u> 1999, vol 107(1), pp 137-142.

1124   Melikian G, et al. "Relation of vitamin A and carotenoid status to growth failure and mortality among ugandan infants with human immunodeficiency virus." <u>Nutrition.</u> 2001, vol 17(7-8), pp 567-572.

1125   Palace VP, et al. "Antioxidant potentials of vitamin A and carotenoids and their relevance to heart disease." <u>Free Radical Biology and Medicine.</u> 1999, vol 26(5-6), pp 746-761.

1126   Omu AE and Fatinikun T. "Significance of simultaneous determination of serum and seminal plasma α-tocopherol and retinol in infertile men by high-performance liquid chromatography." Andrologia. 1999, vol 31(6), pp 347-354.

1127   Bosetti C, et al. "Retinol, carotenoids and the risk of prostate cancer: a case-control study from Italy." Int J Cancer. 2004, vol 112(4), pp 689-692.

1128   Bianchi-Santamaria A, et al. "Short communication: Short communication: Possible activity of beta-carotene in patients with aids related complex. A pilot study." Medical Oncology and Tumor Pharmacotherapy. 1992, vol 9 (3), pp 151-153.

1129   Van Leeuwen R et al. "Dietary Intake of Antioxidants and Risk of Age-Related Macular Degeneration." The Journal of the American Medical Association. 2005, vol 294(24).

1130   Polidori MC, et al. "[Influence of vascular comorbidities on the antioxidant defense system in Alzheimer's disease]." Dtsch Med "Wochenschr. 2012, vol 137(7), pp 305-308.

1131   Tavani A, et al. "Intake of selected micronutrients and the risk of surgically treated benign prostatic hyperplasia: a case-control study from Italy." Eur Urol. 2006, vol 50(3), pp 549-554.

1132   Lee HP et al. "Dietary effects on breast-cancer risk in Singapore." The Lancet. 1991, vol 337(8751), pp 1197-1200.

1133   ST Mayne. "Beta-carotene, carotenoids, and disease prevention in humans." The FASEB Journal. 1996, vol 10(7), pp 690-701.

1134   La Vecchia C et al. "Dietary vitamin A and the risk of invasive cervical cancer." International Journal of Cancer. 1984, vol 34(3), pp 319-322

1135   Muto Y et al. "Growth retardation in human cervical dysplasia-derived cell lines by beta-carotene through down-regulation of epidermal growth factor receptor." Am J Clin Nutr. 1995, vol 62 (6), pp 15355-15405.

1136   Arafa MA, et al. "Dietary and lifestyle characteristics of colorectal cancer in Jordan: a case-control study." Asian Pac J Cancer Prev. 2011, vol 12(8, pp 1931-1936.)

[1137]   Brigitte M et al. "Enhanced resistance to oxidation of low density lipoproteins and decreased lipid peroxide formation during β-carotene supplementation in cystic fibrosis." Free Radical Biology and Medicine. 1995, vol 18(5), pp 849-859.

[1138]   de Oliveira Otto MC, et al. "Dietary intakes of zinc and heme iron from red meat, but not from other sources, are associated with greater risk of metabolic syndrome and cardiovascular disease." J Nutr. 2012, vol 142(3), pp 526-533.

[1139]   Pelucchi C, et al. "Dietary intake of selected micronutrients and gastric cancer risk: an Italian case-control study." Ann Oncol. 2009, vol 20(1), pp 160-165.

[1140]   Coodley GO et al. "Beta-carotene in HIV infection: an extended evaluation." Division of Internal Medicine, Oregon Health Sciences University, Portland 97201-3098, USA. [1996, 10(9):967-973]

Filteau SM, et al. "The Effect of Antenatal Vitamin A and [beta] -Carotene Supplementation on Gut Integrity of Infants of HICV-Infected South African Women." JPGN. 2001, vol 32 (4), pp 464-470.

[1141]   Sommer A. "Nutritional blindness. Xerophthalmia and keratomalacia." Nutritional Blindness. 1982, pp.xiii + 282 pp. ISBN 0-19-502977-1

[1142]   Age-Related Eye Disease Study Research Group. "A randomized, placebo-controlled, clinical trial of high-dose supplementation with vitamins C and E, beta carotene, and zinc for age-related macular degeneration and vision loss: AREDS report no. 8." Arch Ophthalmol. 2001, vol 119(10), pp 1417-1436.

[1143]   Christian P, et al. "Night Blindness During Pregnancy and Subsequent Mortality among Women in Nepal: Effects of Vitamin A and β-Carotene Supplementation." Am J Epidemiol. 2000, 152(6), pp 542-547.

[1144]   Sommer A. "Nutritional blindness. Xerophthalmia and keratomalacia." Nutritional Blindness. 1982, pp.xiii + 282 pp. ISBN 0-19-502977-1

[1145]   Mecca MS, et al. "Ten-week lifestyle changing program reduces several indicators for metabolic syndrome in overweight adults." Diabetol Metab Syndr. 2012, vol 4(1), p 1.

1146   Tsiligianni IG and van der Molen T. "A systematic review of the role of vitamin insufficiencies and supplementation in COPD." <u>Respir Res.</u> 2010, vol 11, p 171.

1147   Ravi F, et al. "Dietary intake of selected micronutrients and the risk of pancreatic cancer: an Italian case-control study." <u>Ann Oncol.</u> 2011, vol 22(1), pp 202-206.

1148   Mathews-Roth MM et al. "Beta Carotene Therapy for Erythropoietic Protoporphyria and Other Photosensitivity Diseases." <u>Arch Dermatol</u>. 1977, vol 113(9), pp 1229-1232.

1149   Seifter E, et al. "Vitamin A Inhibits Some Aspects of Systemic Disease Due to Local X-Radiation." <u>Journal of Potential & Enteral Nutrition</u>. 1981, vol 5(4), pp 288-294.

1150   Barrett-Reis. "Method of Reducing the Risk of Retinopathy of Prematurity in Preterm Infants." US Patent: US 2007/0166354 A1. Pub Date: Jul. 19, 2007.

1151   Bosetti C, et al. "Retinol, carotenoids and the risk of prostate cancer: a case-control study from Italy." <u>Int J Cancer.</u> 2004, vol 112(4), pp 689-692.

1152   Joanne Whitehead. "Intestinal alkaline phosphatase: The molecular link between rosacea and gastrointestinal disease?" <u>Medical Hypotheses</u>. 2009, vol 73(6), pp 1019-1022. http://www.medical-hypotheses.com/article/S0306-9877%2809%2900371-5/abstract

1153   Frieling UM, et al. "A Randomoized, 12-Year Primary_Prevention Trial of Beta Carotene Supplementation from Nonmelanoma Skin Cancer in the Physicaians' Health Study." <u>JAMA Dermatology</u>. 2000, vol 136 (2), pp 179-184. Van Poppel G Goldbohm RA. "Epidemiologic evidence for beta-carotene and cancer prevention." <u>Am J Cliin Nutr</u>. 1995, vol 62(6), pp 1393S-1402S.

1154   Frieling UM, et al. "A Randomoized, 12-Year Primary_Prevention Trial of Beta Carotene Supplementation from Nonmelanoma Skin Cancer in the Physicaians' Health Study." <u>JAMA Dermatology</u>. 2000, vol 136(2), pp 179-184. Van Poppel G Goldbohm RA. "Epidemiologic evidence for beta-carotene and cancer prevention." <u>Am J Clin Nutr</u>. 1995, vol 62(6), pp 1393S-1402S.

1155   Mikhail MS, et al. "Decreased beta-carotene levels in exfoliated vaginal epithelial cells in women with vaginal candidiasis." Am J Reprod Immunol. 1994, vol 32(3), pp 221-225.

1156   Age-Related Eye Disease Study Research Group. "A randomized, placebo-controlled, clinical trial of high-dose supplementation with vitamins C and E, beta carotene, and zinc for age-related macular degeneration and vision loss: AREDS report no. 8." Arch Ophthalmol. 2001, vol 119(10), pp 1417-1436.

1157   Sommer A. "Nutritional blindness. Xerophthalmia and keratomalacia." Nutritional Blindness. 1982, pp.xiii + 282 pp. ISBN 0-19-502977-1

1158   Mecca MS, et al. "Ten-week lifestyle changing program reduces several indicators for metabolic syndrome in overweight adults." Diabetol Metab Syndr. 2012, vol 4(1), p 1.

1159   Hathcock JN. "Vitamin and Mineral Safety, 2nd Edition. Council for Responsible Nutrition (CRN)." 2004.

1160   Ostrea EM, et al. "Influence of breast-feeding on the restoration of the low serum concentration of vitamin E and beta-carotene in the newborn infant." Am J Obstet Gynecol. 1996, vol 154(5), pp 1014-1017.

1161   Frieling UM, et al. "A Randomoized, 12-Year Primary_Prevention Trial of Beta Carotene Supplementation from Nonmelanoma Skin Cancer in the Physicaians' Health Study." JAMA Dermatology. 2000, vol 136 (2), pp 179-184. Van Poppel G Goldbohm RA. "Epidemiologic evidence for beta-carotene and cancer prevention." Am J Cliin Nutr. 1995, vol 62 (6), pp 1393S-1402S.

1162   Virtamo J. "Incidence of cancer and mortality following alpha-tocopherol and beta-carotene supplementation: a postintervention follow-up." Journal of the American Medical Association. 2003. DOI: 10.1001/jama.290.4.476

1163   Christian P, et al. "Night Blindness During Pregnancy and Subsequent Mortality among Women in Nepal: Effects of Vitamin A and β-Carotene Supplementation." Am J Epidemiol. 2000, 152(6), pp 542-547.

1164   http://chemo.net/newpage35.htm

[1165]  Goralczyk R. "Beta-carotene and lung cancer in smokers: review of hypotheses and status of research." <u>Nutr Cancer.</u> 2009, vol 61(6), pp 767-774.

[1166]  Larsson SC, et al. "Dietary carotenoids and risk of hormone receptor-defined breast cancer in a prospective cohort of Swedish women." <u>Eur J Cancer.</u> 2010, vol 46(6), pp 1079-1085.

[1167]  http://lpi.oregonstate.edu/infocenter/phytochemicals/carotenoids/

[1168]  Antioxidants May Help Fight Mesothelioma
Comments OffPosted 22 Feb 2011 — by James Street
Category <u>Antioxidants</u>
Posted on Tuesday, February 22, 2011.
Sources:
Trimmer, Casey at al, "Caveolin-1 and mitochondrial SOD2 (MnSOD) function as tumor suppressors in the stromal microenvironment: A new genetically tractable model for human cancer associated fibroblasts", <u>Cancer Biology & Therapy</u>. February 15, 2011. Volume 11, Issue 4.
"Jefferson Researchers Provide Genetic Evidence that Antioxidants Can Help Treat Cancer", Feb. 15, 2011, <u>Thomas Jefferson University news release</u>, by means of EurekAlert website.
Trimmer, Casey at al, "Caveolin-1 and mitochondrial SOD2 (MnSOD) function as tumor suppressors in the stromal microenvironment: A new genetically tractable model for human cancer associated fibroblasts", <u>Cancer Biology & Therapy.</u> February 15, 2011. Volume 11, Issue 4.
"Jefferson Researchers Provide Genetic Evidence that Antioxidants Can Help Treat Cancer", Feb. 15, 2011, <u>Thomas Jefferson University news release</u>, by way of EurekAlert website.

[1169]  Van Leeuwen R et al. "Dietary Intake of Antioxidants and Risk of Age-Related Macular Degeneration." <u>The Journal of the American Medical Association</u>. 2005, vol 294(24).

[1170]  "Tomatoes, Tomato Based Products, Lycopene, and Cancer: Review of the Epidemiologic Literature ." <u>JNCI J Natl Cancer Inst.</u> 1999, vol 91(4), pp 317-331.

[1171]  Ibid.

[1172]  Ibid..

[1173]  Ibid.

1174   King-Batoon A, et al. "Modulation of gene methylation by genistein or lycopene in breast cancer cells." <u>Environmental and Molecular Mutagenesis.</u> 2008, vol 49(1), pp 36-45.

1175   Gerster H. "The potential role of lycopene for human health." <u>J Am Coll Nutr.</u> 1997, vol 16(2), pp 109-126.

1176   "Tomatoes, Tomato-Based Products, Lycopene, and Cancer: Review of the Epidemiologic Literature ." <u>JNCI J Natl Cancer Inst.</u> 1999, vol 91(4), pp 317-331.

1177   Zini A, et al. "Lycopene supplementation in vitro can protect human sperm deoxyribonucleic acid from oxidative damage." <u>Fertility and Sterility.</u> 2010, vol 94(3), pp 1033-1036.

1178   "Tomatoes, Tomato-Based Products, Lycopene, and Cancer: Review of the Epidemiologic Literature ." <u>JNCI J Natl Cancer Inst.</u> 1999, vol 91(4), pp 317-331.

1179   Barrett-Reis. "Method of Reducing the Risk of Retinopathy of Prematurity in Preterm Infants." US Patent: US 2007/0166354 A1. Pub Date: Jul. 19, 2007.

1180   "Tomatoes, Tomato-Based Products, Lycopene, and Cancer: Review of the Epidemiologic Literature ." <u>JNCI J Natl Cancer Inst.</u> 1999, vol 91(4), pp 317-331.

1181   Cramer DW, et al. "Carotenoids, antioxidants and ovarian cancer risk in pre- and postmenopausal women." <u>International Journal of Cancer.</u> 2001, vol 94(1), pp 128-134.

1182   Giovannucci E, et al. "A Prospective Study of Tomato Products, Lycopene, and Prostate Cancer Risk." <u>JNCI J Natl Cancer Inst.</u> 2000, vol 94(5), pp 391-398.

1183   "Tomatoes, Tomato-Based Products, Lycopene, and Cancer: Review of the Epidemiologic Literature ." <u>JNCI J Natl Cancer Inst.</u> 1999, vol 91(4), pp 317-331.

1184   Ibid.

1185   Ribaya-Mercado JD et al. "Skin Lycopene Is Destroyed Preferentially over ÃŸ-Carotene during ultraviolet Irradiation in Humans1'." <u>Biochemical and Molecular Roles of Nutrients.</u> 1994, pp 1854-1859.

1186   Engelmann NJ, et al. "Nutritional Aspects of Phytoene and Phytofluene, Carotenoid Precursors to Lycopene." Adv Nutr. 2011, vol 2, pp 51-61.

1187   Khachik F, et al. "Chemistry, distribution, and metabolism of tomato carotenoids and their impact on human health." Exp Biol Med (Maywood). 2002, vol 227(10), pp 845-851.

1188   Hirsch K, et al. "Lycopene and other carotenoids inhibit estrogenic activity of 17β-estradiol and genistein in cancer cells." Breast Cancer Research and Treatment. 2007, vol 104(2), pp 221-230.

1189   Liu AG, et al. "Feeding tomato and broccoli powders enriched with bioactives improves bioactivity markers in rats." J Agric Food Chem. 2009, vol 57(16), pp 7304-7310.

1190   Matthew-Roth MM. "PHYTOENE AS A PROTECTIVE AGENT AGAINST SUNBURN (>280nm) RADIATION IN GUINEA PIGS." Photochemistry and Photobiology. 1975, vol 21(4), pp 261-263.

1191   Nishino H, et al. "Carotenoids in Cancer Chemoprevention." Cancer and Metastasis Reviews. 2002, vol 21 (3-4), pp 257-264.

1192   Mathews-Roth MM. "Antitumor Activity of β-Carotene, Canthaxanthin and Phytoene." Oncology. 1982, vol 39(1), pp 33-37.

1193   Stahl W and Sies H. "β-Carotene and other carotenoids in protection from sunlight." Am J Clin Nutr. 2007, vol 96(5), pp 1179S-1184S.

1194   Engelmann NJ, et al. "Nutritional Aspects of Phytoene and Phytofluene, Carotenoid Precursors to Lycopene." Adv Nutr. 2011, vol 2, pp 51-61.

1195   Hirsch K, et al. "Lycopene and other carotenoids inhibit estrogenic activity of 17β-estradiol and genistein in cancer cells." Breast Cancer Research and Treatment. 2007, vol 104(2), pp 221-230.

1196   Aust O, et al. "Supplementation with tomato-based products increases lycopene, phytofluene, and phytoene levels in human serum and protects against UV-light-induced erythema." Int J Vitam Nutr Res. 2005, vol 75(1), pp 54-60.

[1197]   Liu AG, et al. "Feeding tomato and broccoli powders enriched with bioactives improves bioactivity markers in rats." <u>J Agric Food Chem.</u> 2009, vol 57(16), pp 7304-7310.

[1198]   Matthew-Roth MM. "CAROTENOID PIGMENT ADMINISTRATION and DELAY IN DEVELOPMENT OF UV-B-INDUCED TUMORS." <u>Photochemistry and Photobiology.</u> 1983, vol(5), pp 509-511.

[1199]   Stahl W and Sies H. "β-Carotene and other carotenoids in protection from sunlight." <u>Am J Clin Nutr.</u> 2007, vol 96(5), pp 1179S-1184S.

[1200]   Hussein G, et al. "Astaxanthin, a Carotenoid with Potential in Human Health and Nutrition." <u>J Nat Prod.</u> 2006, vol 69(3), pp 443-449.

[1201]   Guerin M, et al. "Haematococcus astaxanthin: applications for human health and
Nutrition." <u>Trends in Biotechnology.</u> 2003, vol 21(5), pp 210-216.

[1202]   Hussein G, et al. "Astaxanthin, a Carotenoid with Potential in Human Health and Nutrition." <u>J Nat Prod.</u> 2006, vol 69(3), pp 443-449.

[1203]   Bob Capelli and Gerald R Cysewski. "Neuroprotective Effects of Astaxanthin." Cyanotech Corp. 2011.

[1204]   Yasushi Nishoika, et al. "The antianxiety-like effect of astaxanthin extracted from *Paracoccus carotinifaciens*." <u>BioFactors.</u> 2011, vol 37(1), pp 25-30.

[1205]   Guerin M, et al. "Haematococcus astaxanthin: applications for human health and
Nutrition." <u>Trends in Biotechnology.</u> 2003, vol 21(5), pp 210-216.

[1206]   Fassett RG and Coombes JS. "Astaxanthin: A Potential Therapeutic Agent in Cardiovascular Disease." <u>Marine Drugs.</u> 2011, vol 9, pp 447-465. doi:10.3390/md9030447.  ISSN 1660-3397

[1207]   Lignell, Ake and Bottiger, Per. "USE OF XANTHOPHYLLS, ASTAXANTHIN E.G., FOR TREATMENT OF AUTOIMMUNE DISEASES, CHRONIC VIRAL AND INTRACELLULAR BACTERIAL INFECTIONS." International Patent Classification A61K 31/122, A61K 31/23, A61P 37/00.  Filed: 2000-10-05.

1208   Chandrasekar B, et al. "Tissue specific regulation of transforming growth factor beta by omega-3 lipid-rich krill oil in autoimmune murine lupus." <u>Nutrition Research.</u> 1996, vol 16(3), pp 489-503.

1209   Guerin M, et al. "Haematococcus astaxanthin: applications for human health and Nutrition." <u>Trends in Biotechnology.</u> 2003, vol 21(5), pp 210-216.

1210   Mark L. Anderson. "A Preliminary Investigation of the Enzymatic Inhibition of 5α-Reductase and Growth of Prostatic Carcinoma Cell Line LNCap-FGC by Natural Astaxanthin and Saw Palmetto Lipid Extract *In Vitro*." <u>Journal of Dietary Supplements.</u> 2005, vol 5(1), pp 17-26.

1211   Hussein G, et al. "Astaxanthin, a Carotenoid with Potential in Human Health and Nutrition." <u>J Nat Prod.</u> 2006, vol 69(3), pp 443-449.

1212   Li Z, et al. "The effects of carotenoids on the proliferation of human breast cancer cell and gene expression of bcl-2." <u>Zhonghua Yu Fang Yi Xue Za Zhi.</u> 2002, vol 36(4), pp 254-257.

1213   Hussein G, et al. "Astaxanthin, a Carotenoid with Potential in Human Health and Nutrition." <u>J Nat Prod.</u> 2006, vol 69(3), pp 443-449.

1214   Fassett RG and Coombes JS. "Astaxanthin: A Potential Therapeutic Agent in Cardiovascular Disease." <u>Marine Drugs.</u> 2011, vol 9, pp 447-465. doi:10.3390/md9030447.  ISSN 1660-3397

1215   Spiller GA, et a. "Effect of daily use natural astaxanthin on C-reactive protein." Health Research & Studies Center, Los Altos CA, 2006, pp 1-6.

1216   Tzu-Hua Wu, et al. "Astaxanthin Protects against Oxidative Stress and Calcium-Induced Porcine Lens Protein Degradation." <u>J Agric Food Chem.</u> 2--6, vol 54(6), pp 2418-2423.

1217   Guerin M, et al. "Haematococcus astaxanthin: applications for human health and Nutrition." <u>Trends in Biotechnology.</u> 2003, vol 21(5), pp 210-216.

1218   Jian-Ping Yuan, et al. "Potential health-promoting effects of astaxanthin: A high-value carotenoid mostly from micro algae." Molecular Nutrition & Food Research. 2010, vol 55(1), pp 150-165.

1219   Katagiri M, et al. "Effects of astaxanthin-rich *Haematococcus pluvialis* extract on cognitive function: a randomised, double-blind, placebo-controlled study." J Clin Biochem Nutr. 2012, vol 51(2), pp 102-107.

1220   Palozza P, et al. "Growth-inhibitory effects of the astaxanthin-rich alga *Haematococcus pluvialis* in human colon cancer cells." Cancer Letters. 2009, vol 283(1), pp 108-117.

1221   Guerin M, et al. "Haematococcus astaxanthin: applications for human health and
Nutrition." Trends in Biotechnology. 2003, vol 21(5), pp 210-216.

1222   Lignell, Ake and Bottiger, Per. "USE OF XANTHOPHYLLS, ASTAXANTHIN E.G., FOR TREATMENT OF AUTOIMMUNE DISEASES, CHRONIC VIRAL AND INTRACELLULAR BACTERIAL INFECTIONS." International Patent Classification A61K 31/122, A61K 31/23, A61P 37/00.  Filed: 2000-10-05.

1223   Hussein G, et al. "Astaxanthin, a Carotenoid with Potential in Human Health and Nutrition." J Nat Prod. 2006, vol 69(3), pp 443-449.

1224   Jian-Ping Yuan, et al. "Potential health-promoting effects of astaxanthin: A high-value carotenoid mostly from micro algae." Molecular Nutrition & Food Research. 2010, vol 55(1), pp 150-165.

1225   Andersen LP, et al. "Gastric inflammatory markers and interleukins in patients with functional dyspepsia treated with astaxanthin." FEMS Immunology & Medical Microbiology. 2007, vol 50(2), pp 244-248.

1226   Guerin M, et al. "Haematococcus astaxanthin: applications for human health and
Nutrition." Trends in Biotechnology. 2003, vol 21(5), pp 210-216.

1227   Yoshimi Nakajimi, et al. "Astaxanthin, a dietary carotenoid, protects retinal cells against oxidative stress in-vitro and in mice in-vivo." Journal of Pharmacy and Pharmacology. 2008, vol 60(10), pp 1365-1374.

[1228]  Jian-Ping Yuan, et al. "Potential health-promoting effects of astaxanthin: A high-value carotenoid mostly from micro algae." Molecular Nutrition & Food Research. 2010, vol 55(1), pp 150-165.

[1229]  Lignell, Ake and Bottiger, Per. "USE OF XANTHOPHYLLS, ASTAXANTHIN E.G., FOR TREATMENT OF AUTOIMMUNE DISEASES, CHRONIC VIRAL AND INTRACELLULAR BACTERIAL INFECTIONS." International Patent Classification A61K 31/122, A61K 31/23, A61P 37/00.  Filed: 2000-10-05.

[1230]  McCarty MF. "Full-spectrum antioxidant therapy featuring astaxanthin coupled with lipoprivic strategies and salsalate for management of non-alcoholic fatty liver disease." Med Hypotheses. 2011, vol 77(4), pp 550-556.

[1231]  Angwafor F 3rd and Anderson ML. "An open label, dose response study to determine the effect of a dietary supplement on dihydrotestosterone, testosterone and estradiol levels in healthy males." J Int Soc Sports Nutr. 2008, vol 5, p 12.

[1232]  Angwafor F 3rd and Anderson ML. "An open label, dose response study to determine the effect of a dietary supplement on dihydrotestosterone, testosterone and estradiol levels in healthy males." J Int Soc Sports Nutr. 2008, vol 5, p 12.

[1233]  Jian-Ping Yuan, et al. "Potential health-promoting effects of astaxanthin: A high-value carotenoid mostly from microalgae." Molecular Nutrition & Food Research. 2011, vol 55(1), pp 150-165.

[1234]  Hussein G, et al. "Astaxanthin, a Carotenoid with Potential in Human Health and Nutrition." J Nat Prod. 2006, vol 69(3), pp 443-449.

[1235]  Ibid.

[1236]  Lignell, Ake and Bottiger, Per. "USE OF XANTHOPHYLLS, ASTAXANTHIN E.G., FOR TREATMENT OF AUTOIMMUNE DISEASES, CHRONIC VIRAL AND INTRACELLULAR BACTERIAL INFECTIONS." International Patent Classification A61K 31/122, A61K 31/23, A61P 37/00.  Filed: 2000-10-05.

[1237]  Fassett RG and Coombes JS. "Astaxanthin: A Potential Therapeutic Agent in Cardiovascular Disease." Marine Drugs. 2011, vol 9, pp 447-465. doi:10.3390/md9030447.  ISSN 1660-3397

1238   Deutsch L. "Evaluation of the Effect of Neptune Krill Oil on Chronic Inflammation and Arthritic Symptoms." J Am Coll Nutr. 2007, vol 26(1), pp 39-48.

1239   Xiaoli Zhang, et al. "Impact of astaxanthin-enriched algal powder of Haematococcus pluvialis on memory improvement in BALB/c mice." Environmental Geochemistry and Health. 2007, vol 29(6), pp 483-489.

1240   Jian-Ping Yuan, et al. "Potential health-promoting effects of astaxanthin: A high-value carotenoid mostly from micro algae." Molecular Nutrition & Food Research. 2010, vol 55(1), pp 150-165.

1241   Guerin M, et al. "Haematococcus astaxanthin: applications for human health and
Nutrition." Trends in Biotechnology. 2003, vol 21(5), pp 210-216.

1242   Jian-Ping Yuan, et al. "Potential health-promoting effects of astaxanthin: A high-value carotenoid mostly from micro algae." Molecular Nutrition & Food Research. 2010, vol 55(1), pp 150-165.

1243   Comhaire FH, et al. "Combined conventional/antioxidant "Astaxanthin" treatment for male infertility: a double blind, randomized trial." Asian J Androl. 2005, vol 7(3), pp 257-262.

1244   Chew BP, et al. "A comparison of the anticancer activities of dietary beta-carotene, canthaxanthin and astaxanthin in mice in vivo." Anticancer Research. 1999, vol 19(3A), pp 1849-1853.

1245   Guerin M, et al. "Haematococcus astaxanthin: applications for human health and Nutrition." Trends in Biotechnology. 2003, vol 21(5), pp 210-216.

1246   Augusti PR, et al. "Effect of astaxanthin on kidney function impairment and oxidative stress induced by mercuric chloride in rats." Food and Chemical Toxicology. 2008, vol 46(1), pp 212-219.

1247   Wolf AM, et al. "Astaxanthin protects mitochondrial redox state and functional integrity against oxidative stress." JNB. 2010, vol 21(5), pp 381-389.

[1248] Lignell, Ake and Bottiger, Per. "USE OF XANTHOPHYLLS, ASTAXANTHIN E.G., FOR TREATMENT OF AUTOIMMUNE DISEASES, CHRONIC VIRAL AND INTRACELLULAR BACTERIAL INFECTIONS." International Patent Classification A61K 31/122, A61K 31/23, A61P 37/00. Filed: 2000-10-05.

[1249] Guerin M, et al. "Haematococcus astaxanthin: applications for human health and Nutrition." Trends in Biotechnology. 2003, vol 21(5), pp 210-216.

[1250] Jeong Hwan Kim, et al. "Astaxanthin improves the proliferative capacity as well as the osteogenic and adipogenic differentiation potential in neural stem cells." Food and Chemical Toxicology. 2010, vol 48(6), pp 1741-1745.

[1251] Guerin M, et al. "Haematococcus astaxanthin: applications for human health and Nutrition." Trends in Biotechnology. 2003, vol 21(5), pp 210-216.

[1252] McCarty MF. "Full-spectrum antioxidant therapy featuring astaxanthin coupled with lipoprivic strategies and salsalate for management of non-alcoholic fatty liver disease." Med Hypotheses. 2011, vol 77(4), pp 550-556.

[1253] Ikeuchi M, et al. "Effects of Astaxanthin in Obese Mice Fed a High-Fat Diet." Bioscience, Biotechnology, and Biochemistry. 2007, vol 71(4), pp 893-899.

[1254] Hussein G, et al. "Astaxanthin, a Carotenoid with Potential in Human Health and Nutrition." J Nat Prod. 2006, vol 69(3), pp 443-449.

[1255] Guerin M, et al. "Haematococcus astaxanthin: applications for human health and Nutrition." Trends in Biotechnology. 2003, vol 21(5), pp 210-216.

[1256] Sampalis F, et al. "Evaluation of the Effects of Neptune Krill Oil on the Management of Premenstrual Syndrome." Altern Med Rev. 2003, vol 8(2), pp 171-179.

[1257] Ibid.

[1258] Hussein G, et al. "Astaxanthin, a Carotenoid with Potential in Human Health and Nutrition." J Nat Prod. 2006, vol 69(3), pp 443-449.

[1259] Guerin M, et al. "Haematococcus astaxanthin: applications for human health and Nutrition." Trends in Biotechnology. 2003, vol 21(5), pp 210-216.

1260   Ibid.

1261   Ibid.

1262  Lignell, Ake and Bottiger, Per. "USE OF XANTHOPHYLLS, ASTAXANTHIN E.G., FOR TREATMENT OF AUTOIMMUNE DISEASES, CHRONIC VIRAL AND INTRACELLULAR BACTERIAL INFECTIONS." International Patent Classification A61K 31/122, A61K 31/23, A61P 37/00.  Filed: 2000-10-05.

1263   Kupcinskas L, et al. "Efficacy of the natural antioxidant astaxanthin in the treatment of functional dyspepsia in patients with or without Helicobacter pylori infection: A prospective, randomized, double blind, and placebo-controlled study." Phytomedicine. 2008, vol 15(6-7).

1264  Lignell, Ake and Bottiger, Per. "USE OF XANTHOPHYLLS, ASTAXANTHIN E.G., FOR TREATMENT OF AUTOIMMUNE DISEASES, CHRONIC VIRAL AND INTRACELLULAR BACTERIAL INFECTIONS." International Patent Classification A61K 31/122, A61K 31/23, A61P 37/00.  Filed: 2000-10-05.

1265   Hussein G, et al. "Astaxanthin, a Carotenoid with Potential in Human Health and Nutrition." J Nat Prod. 2006, vol 69(3), pp 443-449.

1266   Guerin M, et al. "Haematococcus astaxanthin: applications for human health and Nutrition." Trends in Biotechnology. 2003, vol 21(5), pp 210-216.

1267   Jian-Ping Yuan, et al. "Potential health-promoting effects of astaxanthin: A high-value carotenoid mostly from micro algae." Molecular Nutrition & Food Research. 2010, vol 55(1), pp 150-165.

1268   Guerin M, et al. "Haematococcus astaxanthin: applications for human health and Nutrition." Trends in Biotechnology. 2003, vol 21(5), pp 210-216.

1269   Hussein G, et al. "Astaxanthin, a Carotenoid with Potential in Human Health and Nutrition." J Nat Prod. 2006, vol 69(3), pp 443-449.

1270   Fassett RG and Coombes JS. "Astaxanthin: A Potential Therapeutic Agent in Cardiovascular Disease." Marine Drugs. 2011, vol 9, pp 447-465. doi:10.3390/md9030447.  ISSN 1660-3397

1271  Lignell, Ake and Bottiger, Per. "USE OF XANTHOPHYLLS, ASTAXANTHIN E.G., FOR TREATMENT OF AUTOIMMUNE DISEASES, CHRONIC VIRAL AND INTRACELLULAR BACTERIAL INFECTIONS." International Patent Classification A61K 31/122, A61K 31/23, A61P 37/00.  Filed: 2000-10-05.

1272  Hussein G, et al. "Astaxanthin, a Carotenoid with Potential in Human Health and Nutrition." J Nat Prod. 2006, vol 69(3), pp 443-449.

1273  Lignell, Ake and Bottiger, Per. "USE OF XANTHOPHYLLS, ASTAXANTHIN E.G., FOR TREATMENT OF AUTOIMMUNE DISEASES, CHRONIC VIRAL AND INTRACELLULAR BACTERIAL INFECTIONS." International Patent Classification A61K 31/122, A61K 31/23, A61P 37/00.  Filed: 2000-10-05.

1274  Guerin M, et al. "Haematococcus astaxanthin: applications for human health and Nutrition." Trends in Biotechnology. 2003, vol 21(5), pp 210-216.

1275  Camera E, et al. "Astaxanthin, canthaxanthin and beta-carotene differently affect UVA-induced oxidative damage and expression of oxidative stress-responsive enzymes." Exp Dermatol. 2009, vol 18(3), pp 222-231.

1276  Guerin M, et al. "Haematococcus astaxanthin: applications for human health and Nutrition." Trends in Biotechnology. 2003, vol 21(5), pp 210-216.

1277  Ibid.

1278  Hussein G, et al. "Astaxanthin, a Carotenoid with Potential in Human Health and Nutrition." J Nat Prod. 2006, vol 69(3), pp 443-449.

1279  Guerin M, et al. "Haematococcus astaxanthin: applications for human health and Nutrition." Trends in Biotechnology. 2003, vol 21(5), pp 210-216.

1280  Hussein G, et al. "Astaxanthin, a Carotenoid with Potential in Human Health and Nutrition." J Nat Prod. 2006, vol 69(3), pp 443-449.

1281  Ibid.

1282  Ibid.

[1283]   Chew BP, et al. "A comparison of the anticancer activities of dietary beta-carotene, canthaxanthin and astaxanthin in mice in vivo." Anticancer Research. 1999, vol 19(3A), pp 1849-1853.

[1284]   Hussein G, et al. "Astaxanthin, a Carotenoid with Potential in Human Health and Nutrition." J Nat Prod. 2006, vol 69(3), pp 443-449.

[1285]   Guerin M, et al. "Haematococcus astaxanthin: applications for human health and Nutrition." Trends in Biotechnology. 2003, vol 21(5), pp 210-216.

[1286]   Hussein G, et al. "Astaxanthin, a Carotenoid with Potential in Human Health and Nutrition." J Nat Prod. 2006, vol 69(3), pp 443-449.

[1287]   Suzuki K, et al. "Association of abdominal obesity with decreased serum levels of carotenoids in a healthy Japanese population." Clin Nutr. 2006, vol 25(5), pp 780-789.

[1288]   Masanori, et al. "A nerve-regenerating agent comprising, as an active ingredient, arachidonic acid and/or a compound containing arachidonic acid as a constituent fatty acid." European Patent Application: EP2098229.  Application Number: EP20070860598  Date: 12/27/2007.

[1289]   Tina Sampalis. "KRILL EXTRACTS FOR PREVENTION AND/OR TREATMENT OF CARDIOVASCULAR DISEASES." European Patent EP1406641 B1. Date: 01/07/2002.

[1290]   Murillo E. "Hypercholesterolemic effect of canthaxanthin and astaxanthin in rats." Archivos Latinoamericanos de Nutricion. 1992, vol 42(4), pp 409-413.

[1291]   Chew BP, et al. "A comparison of the anticancer activities of dietary beta-carotene, canthaxanthin and astaxanthin in mice in vivo." Anticancer Research. 1999, vol 19(3A), pp 1849-1853.

[1292]   Kung-chi Chan, et al. "Antioxidative and Anti-Inflammatory Neuroprotective Effects of Astaxanthin and Canthaxanthin in Nerve Growth Factor Differentiated PC12 Cells." Journal of Food Science. 2009, vol 74(7), pp H225-H231.

[1293]   Masanori, et al. "A nerve-regenerating agent comprising, as an active ingredient, arachidonic acid and/or a compound containing arachidonic acid as a constituent fatty acid." European Patent Application: EP2098229.  Application Number: EP20070860598  Date: 12/27/2007.

1294  Kumaresan N, et al. "Partially saturated canthaxanthin purified from Aspergillus carbonarius induces apoptosis in prostrate cancer cell line." <u>Appl Microbiol Biotechnol.</u> 2008, vol 80(3), pp 467-473.

1295  Camera E, et al. "Astaxanthin, canthaxanthin and beta-carotene differently affect UVA-induced oxidative damage and expression of oxidative stress-responsive enzymes." <u>Exp Dermatol.</u> 2009, vol 18(3), pp 222-231.

1296  Chew BP, et al. "A comparison of the anticancer activities of dietary beta-carotene, canthaxanthin and astaxanthin in mice in vivo." Anticancer Research. 1999, vol 19(3A), pp 1849-1853.

1297  Bluhm R, et al. "Aplastic Anemia Associated With Canthaxanthin Ingested for 'Tanning' Purposes." <u>JAMA.</u> 1990, vol 264(9), pp 1141-1142.

1298  Rinaldi P, et al. "Plasma antioxidants are similarly depleted in mild cognitive impairment and in Alzheimer's disease." <u>Neurobiology of Aging.</u> 2003, vol 24(7), pp 915-919.

1299  Tamimi RM, et al. "Circulating carotenoids, mammographic density, and subsequent risk of breast cancer." <u>Cancer Res.</u> 2009, vol 69(24), pp 9323-9329.

1300  Irwig MS, et al. "Frequent Intake of Tropical Fruits That Are Rich in β-Cryptoxanthin Is Associated with Higher Plasma β-Cryptoxanthin Concentrations in Costa Rican Adolescents." <u>J Nutr.</u> 2002, vol 132(10), pp 3161-3167.

1301  Ibid.

1302  Tanaka T, et al. "Suppression of azoxymethane-induced colon carcinogenesis in male F344 rats by mandarin juices rich in β-cryptoxanthin and hesperidin." <u>International Journal of Cancer.</u> 2000, vol 88(1), pp 146-150.

1303  Lidebjer C, et al. "Low plasma levels of oxygenated carotenoids in patients with coronary artery disease." <u>Nutr Metab Cardiovasc Dis.</u> 2007, vol 17(6), pp 448-456.

1304  Rinaldi P, et al. "Plasma antioxidants are similarly depleted in mild cognitive impairment and in Alzheimer's disease." <u>Neurobiology of Aging.</u> 2003, vol 24(7), pp 915-919.

[1305]  Montonen J, et al. "Dietary Antioxidant Intake and Risk of Type 2 Diabetes." <u>AMA Diabetes Care.</u> 2004, vol 27(2), pp362-366.

[1306]  Melikian G, et al. "Relation of vitamin A and carotenoid status to growth failure and mortality among ugandan infants with human immunodeficiency virus." <u>Nutrition.</u> 2001, vol 17(7-8), pp 567-572.

[1307]  Pattison DJ, et al. "Dietary β-cryptoxanthin and inflammatory polyarthritis: results from a population-based prospective study." <u>Am J Clin Nutr.</u> 2005, vol 82(2), pp 451-455.

[1308]  Holick CN, et al. "Dietary Carotenoids, Serum β-Carotene, and Retinol and Risk of Lung Cancer in the Alpha-Tocopherol, Beta-Carotene Cohort Study." <u>Am J Epidemiol.</u> 2002, vol 156(6), pp 536-547.

[1309]  Kohno H, et al. "Inhibitory effect of mandarin juice rich in beta-cryptoxanthin and hesperidin on 4-(methylnitrosamino)-1-(3-pyridyl)-1-butanone-induced pulmonary tumorigenesis in mice." <u>Cancer Lett.</u> 2001, vol 174(2), pp 141-150.

[1310]  Yulin Li, et al. "Intakes of selected food groups and beverages and adult acute myeloid leukemia." Leukemia Research. 2006, vol 30(12), pp 1507-1515.

[1311]  Chiu BC, et al. "Dietary intake of fruit and vegetables and risk of non-Hodgkin lymphoma." <u>Cancer Causes Control.</u> 2011, vol 22(8), pp 1183-1195.

[1312]  Brock KE, et al. "Fruit, vegetables, fibre and micronutrients and risk of US renal cell carcinoma." <u>Br J Nutr.</u> 2012, vol 108(6), pp 1077-1085.

[1313]  Pattison DJ, et al. "Dietary β-cryptoxanthin and inflammatory polyarthritis: results from a population-based prospective study." <u>Am J Clin Nutr.</u> 2005, vol 82(2), pp 451-455.

[1314]  Gale CR, et al. "Lutein and Zeaxanthin Status and Risk of Age-Related Macular Degeneration." <u>Invest Ophthalmol.</u> 2003, vol 44(6), pp 2461-2465.

[1315]  Wei Wang, et al. "Nutritional Biomarkers in Alzheimer's Disease: The Association between Carotenoids, n-3 Fatty Acids, and Dementia Severity ." <u>Journal of Alzheimer's Disease.</u> 2008, vol 13(13), pp 31-38.

[1316]   Lidebjer C, et al. "Low plasma levels of oxygenated carotenoids in patients with coronary artery disease." <u>Nutr Metab Cardiovasc Dis.</u> 2007, vol 17(6), pp 448-456.

[1317]   Mares-Perlman JA, et al. "The Body of Evidence to Support a Protective Role for Lutein and Zeaxanthin in Delaying Chronic Disease. Overview." <u>J Nutr.</u> 2002, vol 132(3), pp 518S-524S.

[1318]   Mares-Perlman JA, et al. "The Body of Evidence to Support a Protective Role for Lutein and Zeaxanthin in Delaying Chronic Disease. Overview." <u>J Nutr.</u> 2002, vol 132(2), pp 518S-524S.

[1319]   Slattery ML, et al. "Carotenoids and colon cancer." <u>Am J Clin Nutr.</u> 2000, vol 71(2), pp 575-582.

[1320]   Ibid.

[1321]   Lidebjer C, et al. "Low plasma levels of oxygenated carotenoids in patients with coronary artery disease." <u>Nutr Metab Cardiovasc Dis.</u> 2007, vol 17(6), pp 448-456.

[1322]   Sasaki M, et al. "Neurodegenerative influence of oxidative stress in the retina of a murine model of diabetes." <u>Diabetologia.</u> 2010, vol 53(5), pp 971-979.

[1323]   Neacşu A, et al. "Neuroprotection with carotenoids in glaucoma." <u>Oftalmologia.</u> 2003, vol 59(4), pp 70-75,

[1324]   Melikian G, et al. "Relation of vitamin A and carotenoid status to growth failure and mortality among ugandan infants with human immunodeficiency virus." <u>Nutrition.</u> 2001, vol 17(7-8), pp 567-572.

[1325]   Holick CN, et al. "Dietary Carotenoids, Serum $\beta$-Carotene, and Retinol and Risk of Lung Cancer in the Alpha-Tocopherol, Beta-Carotene Cohort Study." <u>Am J Epidemiol.</u> 2002, vol 156(6), pp 536-547.

[1326]   Nkondjock A, et al. "Dietary Intake of Lycopene Is Associated with Reduced Pancreatic Cancer Risk." <u>J Nutr.</u> 2005, vol 135(3), pp 592-597.

[1327]  Johnson CC, et al. "Adult nutrient intake as a risk factor for Parkinson's disease." <u>Int J Epidemiol.</u> 1999, vol 28(6), pp 1102-1109.

[1328]  Stringham JM, et al. "The Influence of Dietary Lutein and Zeaxanthin on Visual Performance." <u>Journal of Food Science.</u> 2010, vol 75(1), pp R24-R29.

[1329]  Zhang S, et al. "Dietary Carotenoids and Vitamins A, C, and E and Risk of Breast Cancer." <u>JNCI.</u> 1999, vol 91(6), pp 547-556.

[1330]  Stringham JM, et al. "The Influence of Dietary Lutein and Zeaxanthin on Visual Performance." <u>Journal of Food Science.</u> 2010, vol 75(1), pp R24-R29.

[1331]  Steinmetz KA and Potter JD. "Vegetables, fruit, and cancer prevention: a review." <u>Journal of American Dietetic Association.</u> 1996, vol 96(10), pp 1027-1039.

[1332]  Khachik F, et al. "Lutein, lycopene, and their oxidative metabolites in chemoprevention of cancer." <u>Journal of Cellular Biochemistry.</u> 1995, vol 59(22), pp 236-246.

[1333]  Beatty S, et al. The role of oxidative stress in the pathogenesis of age-related macular degeneration. Survey of Ophthalmology. 2000, vol 45 (2), pp 115-134.

[1334]  Wei Wang, et al. "Nutritional Biomarkers in Alzheimer's Disease: The Association between Carotenoids, n-3 Fatty Acids, and Dementia Severity." <u>Journal of Alzheimer's Disease.</u> 2008, vol 13(1), 31-38.

[1335]  Dwyer JH, et al. Progression of Carotid Intima-Media Thickness and Plasma Antioxidants: The Los Angeles Atherosclerosis Study. Arterioxclerosis, Thrombosis, and Vascular Biology. 2004, vol 24, pp 313-319.

[1336]  Li Z, et al. "The effects of carotenoids on the proliferation of human breast cancer cell and gene expression of bcl-2." <u>Zhonghua Yu Fang Yi Xue Za Zhi.</u> 2002, vol 36(4), pp 254-257.

[1337]  Mares-Perlman JA, et al. "The Body of Evidence to Support a Protective Role for Lutein and Zeaxanthin in Delaying Chronic Disease. Overview." <u>J Nutr.</u> 2002, vol 132(2), pp 518S-524S.

[1338]   Gale CR, et al. "Lutein and Zeaxanthin Status and Risk of Age-Related Macular Degeneration." <u>Invest Ophthalmol.</u> 2003, vol 44(6), pp 2461-2465.

[1339]   Wei Wang, et al. "Nutritional Biomarkers in Alzheimer's Disease: The Association between Carotenoids, n-3 Fatty Acids, and Dementia Severity." <u>Journal of Alzheimer's Disease.</u> 2008, vol 13(1), 31-38.

[1340]   Kowluru RA, et al. "Beneficial Effect of Zeaxanthin on Retinal Metabolic Abnormalities in Diabetic Rats." <u>Invest Ophthalmol Vis Sci.</u> 2008, vol 49(4), pp 1645-1651.

[1341]   Neacşu A, et al. "Neuroprotection with carotenoids in glaucoma." <u>Oftalmologia.</u> 2003, vol 59(4), pp 70-75,

[1342]   Melikian G, et al. "Relation of vitamin A and carotenoid status to growth failure and mortality among ugandan infants with human immunodeficiency virus." <u>Nutrition.</u> 2001, vol 17(7-8), pp 567-572.

[1343]   Neacşu A, et al. "Neuroprotection with carotenoids in glaucoma." <u>Oftalmologia.</u> 2003, vol 59(4), pp 70-75,

[1344]   Holick CN, et al. "Dietary Carotenoids, Serum $\beta$-Carotene, and Retinol and Risk of Lung Cancer in the Alpha-Tocopherol, Beta-Carotene Cohort Study." <u>Am J Epidemiol.</u> 2002, vol 156(6), pp 536-547.

[1345]   Stringham JM, et al. "The Influence of Dietary Lutein and Zeaxanthin on Visual Performance." <u>Journal of Food Science.</u> 2010, vol 75(1), pp R24-R29.

[1346]   Zhang S, et al. "Dietary Carotenoids and Vitamins A, C, and E and Risk of Breast Cancer." <u>JNCI.</u> 1999, vol 91(6), pp 547-556.

[1347]   Barrett-Reis. "Method of Reducing the Risk of Retinopathy of Prematurity in Preterm Infants." US Patent: US 2007/0166354 A1. Pub Date: Jul. 19, 2007.

[1348]   Stringham JM, et al. "The Influence of Dietary Lutein and Zeaxanthin on Visual Performance." <u>Journal of Food Science.</u> 2010, vol 75(1), pp R24-R29.

[1349]   Maccarrone M, et al. The Photoreceptor Protector Zeaxanthin Induces Cell Death in Neuroblastoma Cells. Anticancer Research. 2005, vol 25 (6B), pp 3871-3876.

[1350]   Zhen Sun, and Huiyuan Yao. The influence of di-acetylation of the hydroxyl groups on the anti-tumor-proliferation activity of lutein and zeaxanthin. <u>Asia Pac J Clin Nutr.</u> 2007, vol 16 (1), pp 447-452.

[1351]   Novak E. "Method of Preventing and Delaying onset of Alzheimer's Disease and Composition Therefor." US Patent 5,985,936. Date: Nov 16, 1999.

[1352]   Farquhar JW, et al. "The Effect of Beta Sitosterol on the Serum Lipids of Young Men with Arteriosclerotic Heart Disease." <u>Circulation.</u> 1956, vol 14, pp 77-82.

[1353]   Alappat L, et al. "Effect of vitamin D and β-sitosterol on immune function of macrophages." <u>International Immunopharmacology.</u> 2010, vol 10(11), pp 1390-1396.

[1354]   Nahata A and Dixit VK. "Ameliorative effects of stinging nettle (Urtica dioica) on testosterone-induced prostatic hyperplasia in rats." <u>Andrologia.</u> 2012, vol 44(1), pp 396-409.

[1355]   Awad AB, et al. "Inhibition of growth and stimulation of apoptosis by beta-sitosterol treatment of MDA-MB-231 human breast cancer cells in culture." <u>Int J Mol Med.</u> 2000, vol 5(5), pp 541-545.

[1356]   Jones PJH and AbuMweis SS. "Phytosterols as functional food ingredients: linkages to cardiovascular disease and cancer." <u>Current Opinion in Clinical Nutrition & Metabolic Care.</u> 2009, vol 12(2), pp 147-151.

[1357]   Ibid.

[1358]   Fergusson A and Davidson JC. "COMPOSITION FOR THE REGULATION OF THE HUMAN IMMUNE SYSTEM AND THE PREVENTION AND TREATMENT OF DISEASE THEREOF." Patent US2005/0182037 A1.  Date: Aug 18, 2005.

[1359]   Choi YH, et al. "Induction of Bax and activation of caspases during beta-sitosterol-mediated apoptosis in human colon cancer cells." <u>International Journal of Oncology.</u> 2003, vol 23(6), pp 1657-1662.

[1360]  Fergusson A and Davidson JC. "COMPOSITION FOR THE REGULATION OF THE HUMAN IMMUNE SYSTEM AND THE PREVENTION AND TREATMENT OF DISEASE THEREOF." Patent US2005/0182037 A1.  Date: Aug 18, 2005.

[1361]  Ibid.

[1362]  Ibid.

[1363]  Olalde Rangel, JA. "Synergistic HIV/AIDS and/or IMMUNE DISEASE PHYTO-NUTRACEUTICAL COMPOSITION." US Patent US 7,604,823 B2. Date: Oct 20, 2009.

[1364]  Fergusson A and Davidson JC. "COMPOSITION FOR THE REGULATION OF THE HUMAN IMMUNE SYSTEM AND THE PREVENTION AND TREATMENT OF DISEASE THEREOF." Patent US2005/0182037 A1.  Date: Aug 18, 2005.

[1365]  Ibid.

[1366]  Ibid.

[1367]  Park C, et al. "Beta-sitosterol induces anti-proliferation and apoptosis in human leukemic U937 cells through activation of caspase-3 and induction of Bax/Bcl-2 ratio." Biol Pharm Bull. 2007(7), 1317-1323.

[1368]  Fergusson A and Davidson JC. "COMPOSITION FOR THE REGULATION OF THE HUMAN IMMUNE SYSTEM AND THE PREVENTION AND TREATMENT OF DISEASE THEREOF." Patent US2005/0182037 A1.  Date: Aug 18, 2005.

[1369]  Ibid.

[1370]  von Holtz RL, et al. "beta-Sitosterol activates the sphingomyelin cycle and induces apoptosis in LNCaP human prostate cancer cells." Nutr Cancer. 1998, vol 32(1), pp 8-12.

[1371]  Zhao Y, et al. "Beta-sitosterol inhibits cell growth and induces apoptosis in SGC-7901 human stomach cancer cells." J Agric Food Chem. 2009, vol 57(12), pp 5211-3218.

1372   Donald PR, et al. "A randomised placebo-controlled trial of the efficacy of beta-sitosterol and its glucoside as adjuvants in the treatment of pulmonary tuberculosis." The International Journal of Tuberculosis and Lung Disease. 1997, vol 1(6), pp 518-522(5).

1373   Heverin M, et al. "Changes in the levels of cerebral and extracerebral sterols in the brain of patients with Alzheimer's disease." Journal of Lipid Research. 2004, vol 45, pp 186-193.

1374   Hsu HF, et al. "Typhonium blumei extract inhibits proliferation of human lung adenocarcinoma A549 cells via induction of cell cycle arrest and apoptosis." J Ethnopharmacol. 2011, vol 135(2)pp 492-500.

1375   Genser B, et al. "Plant sterols and cardiovascular disease: a systematic review and meta-analysis." Eur Heart J. 2012, vol 33(4), pp 444-451.

1376   Gabay O, et al. "Stigmasterol: a phytosterol with potential anti-osteoarthritic properties." Osteoarthritis and Cartilage. 2010, vol 18(1), pp 106-116.

1377   Awad AB and Fink CS. "Phytosterols as Anticancer Dietary Components: Evidence and Mechanism of Action." J Nutr. 2000, vol 130(9), pp 2127-2130.

1378   Gylling H and Miettinen TA. "The effect of plant stanol- and sterol-enriched foods on lipid metabolism, serum lipids and coronary heart disease." Ann Clin Biochem. 2005, vol 42(4), pp 254-263.

1379   Hsu HF, et al. "Typhonium blumei extract inhibits proliferation of human lung adenocarcinoma A549 cells via induction of cell cycle arrest and apoptosis." J Ethnopharmacol. 2011, vol 135(2)pp 492-500.

1380   Leichtle AB, et al. "Effects of a 2-y dietary weight-loss intervention on cholesterol metabolism in moderately obese men." Am J Clin Nutr. 2011, vol 94(5), pp 1189-1195.

1381   Hsu HF, et al. "Typhonium blumei extract inhibits proliferation of human lung adenocarcinoma A549 cells via induction of cell cycle arrest and apoptosis." J Ethnopharmacol. 2011, vol 135(2)pp 492-500.

[1382]   Hsu HF, et al. "Typhonium blumei extract inhibits proliferation of human lung adenocarcinoma A549 cells via induction of cell cycle arrest and apoptosis." J Ethnopharmacol. 2011, vol 135(2)pp 492-500.

[1383]   Hsu HF, et al. "Typhonium blumei extract inhibits proliferation of human lung adenocarcinoma A549 cells via induction of cell cycle arrest and apoptosis." J Ethnopharmacol. 2011, vol 135(2)pp 492-500.

[1384]   Hsu HF, et al. "Typhonium blumei extract inhibits proliferation of human lung adenocarcinoma A549 cells via induction of cell cycle arrest and apoptosis." J Ethnopharmacol. 2011, vol 135(2)pp 492-500.

[1385]   Grimm OW, et al. "Stigmasterol For the Treatment of Alzheimer's Disease." International Application: PCT/NL2010/050133. Date: 12.03.2010

[1386]   Moghadasian MH and Frohlich JJ. "Effects of dietary phytosterols on cholesterol metabolism and atherosclerosis: clinical and experimental evidence." American Journal of Medicine. 1999, vol 107(6), pp 588-594.

[1387]   Awad AB and Fink CS. "Phytosterols as Anticancer Dietary Components: Evidence and Mechanism of Action." J Nutr. 2000, vol 130(9), pp 2127-2130.

[1388]   Ryan E, et al. "Fatty acid profile, tocopherol, squalene and phytosterol content of brazil, pecan, pine, pistachio and cashew nuts." International Journal of Food Sciences and Nutrition. 2006, vol 57(3-4), pp 219-228.

[1389]   Awad AB and Fink CS. "Phytosterols as Anticancer Dietary Components: Evidence and Mechanism of Action." J Nutr. 2000, vol 130(9), pp 2127-2130.

[1390]   Gabay O, et al. "Stigmasterol: a phytosterol with potential anti-osteoarthritic properties." Osteoarthritis Cartilage. 2010, vol 18(1), pp 106-116.

[1391]   Valerio M, et al. "Phytosterols ameliorate clinical manifestations and inflammation in experimental autoimmune encephalomyelitis." Inflammation Research. 2011, vol 60(5), pp 457-465.

[1392]   Strom SS, et al. "Phytoestrogen intake and prostate cancer: A case-control study using a new database." Nutrition and Cander. 1999, vol 33(1), pp 20-25.

1393   Gabay O, et al. "Stigmasterol: a phytosterol with potential anti-osteoarthritic properties." <u>Osteoarthritis Cartilage.</u> 2010, vol 18(1), pp 106-116.

1394   da Silva ML, et al. "Anti-snake venom activities of extracts and fractions from callus cultures of Sapindus saponaria." <u>Pharm Biol.</u> 2012, vol 50(3), pp 366-375.

1395   Ibid.

1396   Takayuki Sugiura, et al. "Lysophosphatidic acid, a growth factor-like lipid,in the saliva." <u>ASBMB Journal of Lipid Research.</u> 2002, vol 43, pp 2049-2055.

1397   Di Paolo G and Tae-Wan Kim. "Linking lipids to Alzheimer's disease: cholesterol and beyond." <u>Nature Reviews Neuroscience.</u> 2011, vol 12, pp 284-296.

1398   Siess W, et al. "Lysophosphatidic acid mediates the rapid activation of platelets and endothelial cells by mildly oxidized low density lipoprotein and accumulates in human atherosclerotic lesions." <u>Proc Natl Acad Sci USA.</u> 1999, vol 96(12), pp 6931-6936.

1399   Rother E, et al. "Subtype-Selective Antagonists of Lysophosphatidic Acid Receptors Inhibit Platelet Activation Triggered by the Lipid Core of Atherosclerotic Plaques." <u>Circulation.</u> 2003, vol 108, pp 741-747.

1400   Y Xu, et al. "Lysophospholipids activate ovarian and breast cancer cells." <u>Biochem J.</u> 1995, vol 309(Pt 3), pp 933-940.

1401   Mills GB and Moolenaar WH. "The emerging role of lysophosphatidic acid in cancer." <u>Nature Reviews Cancer.</u> 2003, vol 3, pp 582-591.

1402   Lin ME, et al. "Lysophosphatidic acid (LPA) receptors: signaling properties and disease relevance." <u>Prostaglandins Other Lipid Mediat.</u> 2010, vol 91(3-4), pp 130-138.

1403   Ibid.

1404   Nadra K, et al. "Phosphatidic acid mediates demyelination in *Lpin1* mutant mice." <u>Genes & Dev.</u> 2008, vol 22, pp 1647-1661.

1405   Choi JW, et al. "LPA receptors: subtypes and biological actions." <u>Annu Rev Pharmacol Toxicol.</u> 2010, vol 50, pp 157-186.

1406   Ibid.

1407   Clayton DF and George JM. "Synucleins in synaptic plasticity and neurodegenerative disorders." <u>Journal of Neuroscience Research.</u> 1999, vol 58(1), pp 120-129.

1408   Lin ME, et al. "Lysophosphatidic acid (LPA) receptors: signaling properties and disease relevance." <u>Prostaglandins Other Lipid Mediat.</u> 2010, vol 91(3-4), pp 130-138.

1409   Ibid.

1410   Ulrix W, et al. "Identification of the Phosphatidic Acid Phosphatase Type 2a Isozyme as an Androgen-regulated Gene in the Human Prostatic Adenocarcinoma Cell Line LNCaP." <u>Journal of Biological Chemistry.</u> 1998, vol 273, pp 4660-4665.

1411   Lin ME, et al. "Lysophosphatidic acid (LPA) receptors: signaling properties and disease relevance." <u>Prostaglandins Other Lipid Mediat.</u> 2010, vol 91(3-4), pp 130-138.

1412   Takayuki Sugiura, et al. "Lysophosphatidic acid, a growth factor-like lipid,in the saliva." <u>ASBMB Journal of Lipid Research.</u> 2002, vol 43, pp 2049-2055.

1413   Wang X, et al. "Signaling functions of phosphatidic acid." <u>Progress in Lipid Research.</u> 2006, vol 45(3), pp 250-278.

1414   Moolenaar WH, et al. "Growth factor-like action of phosphatidic acid." <u>Nature.</u>1986, vol 323, pp 171-173.

1415   Billah MM, et al. "Phospholipase Az Activity Specific for Phosphatidic Acid." <u>Journal of Biological Chemistry.</u> 1981, vol 256(11), pp 5399-5403.

1416   Nadra K, et al. "Phosphatidic acid mediates demyelination in *Lpin1* mutant mice." <u>Genes & Dev.</u> 2008, vol 22, pp 1647-1661.

1417   Clayton DF and George JM. "Synucleins in synaptic plasticity and neurodegenerative disorders." <u>Journal of Neuroscience Research.</u> 1999, vol 58(1), pp 120-129.

1418   Lin ME, et al. "Lysophosphatidic acid (LPA) receptors: signaling properties and disease relevance." Prostaglandins Other Lipid Mediat. 2010, vol 91(3-4), pp 130-138.

1419   Ibid.

1420   Teo ST, et al. "Lysophosphatidic acid in vascular development and disease." IUBMB Life. 2009, vol 61(8), pp 791-799.

1421   Liever CS, et al. "Attenuation of alcohol-induced hepatic fibrosis by polyunsaturated lecithin." Hepatology. 1990, vol 12(6), pp 1390-1398.

1422   Soderberg M, et al. "Fatty acid composition of brain phospholipids in aging and in Alzheimer's disease." Lipids. 1991, vol 26(6), pp 421-425.

1423   Stoll AL, et al. "Choline in the treatment of rapid-cycling bipolar disorder: Clinical and neurochemical findings in lithium-treated patients." Biological Psychiatry. 1996, vol 40(5), pp 382-388.

1424   Liever CS, et al. "Attenuation of alcohol-induced hepatic fibrosis by polyunsaturated lecithin." Hepatology. 1990, vol 12(6), pp 1390-1398.

1425   Barbeau A. "Emerging treatments: replacement therapy with choline or lecithin in neurological diseases." The Canadian Journal of Neurological Sciences. 1978, vol 51), pp 157-160.

1426   Calandra S, et al."Plasma Lecithin: Cholesterol Acyltransferase Activity in Liver Disease." European Journal of Clinical Investigation. 1971, vol 1(5), pp 352-360.

1427   Barbeau A. "Emerging treatments: replacement therapy with choline or lecithin in neurological diseases." The Canadian Journal of Neurological Sciences. 1978, vol 51), pp 157-160.

1428   Chan H, Abraham G, and Oreopoulos DG. "Oral lecithin improves ultrafiltration in patients on peritoneal dialysis." Perit Dial Int. 1989, vol 9(3), pp 203-205.

1429   Calandra S, et al."Plasma Lecithin: Cholesterol Acyltransferase Activity in Liver Disease." <u>European Journal of Clinical Investigation.</u> 1971, vol 1(5), pp 352-360.

1430   Lieber CS, et al. "Phosphatidylcholine protects against fibrosis and cirrhosis in the baboon." <u>Gastrroenterology.</u> 1994, vol 106(1), pp 152-159.

1431   Shaw GM, et al. "Choline and Risk of Neural Tube Defects in a Folate-fortified Population." <u>Epidemiology.</u> 2009, vol 20(5), pp 714-719.

1432  Hirsch AR.  "Use of lecithin to restore olfaction and taste." Europen Patent: EP0389667 A2. Date: 10-03-1990.

1433   Ross BM, et al. "Low activity of key phospholipid catabolic and anabolic enzymes in human substantia nigra: possible implications for Parkinson's disease." <u>Neuroscience.</u> 1998, vol 83(3), pp 791-798.

1434   Barbeau A. "Emerging treatments: replacement therapy with choline or lecithin in neurological diseases." <u>The Canadian Journal of Neurological Sciences.</u> 1978, vol 51), pp 157-160.

1435   Deutsch, et al. "First Administration of Cytidine Diphosphocholine and Galantamine in Schizophrenia: A Sustained [alpha]7 Nicotinic Agonist Strategy." 2008, vol 31(1), pp 34-39.

1436   "Treatment of tardive duskiness with lecithin." <u>American Journal of psychiatry.</u> 1979, vol 136, pp 1458-1460.

1437   Barbeau A. "Emerging treatments: replacement therapy with choline or lecithin in neurological diseases." <u>The Canadian Journal of Neurological Sciences.</u> 1978, vol 51), pp 157-160.

1438   Shaw GM, et al. "Choline and Risk of Neural Tube Defects in a Folate-fortified Population." <u>Epidemiology.</u> 2009, vol 20(5), pp 714-719.

1439   McCleary EL. "COMPOSITION AND METHOD FOR TREATING IMPAIRED OR DETERIORATING NEUROLOGICAL FUNCTION." Patent: US 6,964,969 B2. Date: Nov 15, 2005.

1440 Funfgeld EW, et al. "Double-blind study with phosphatidylserine (PS) in parkinsonian patients with senile dementia of Alzheimer's type (SDAT)." <u>Prog Clin Biol Res.</u> 1989, pp 1235-1246.

1441 Peale PK. "COMPOSITION OF PYRUVATE AND ANTICORTISOL COMPOUNDS AND METHOD FOR INCREASING PROTEIN CONCENTRATION IN A MAMMAL." Patent: 5,756,469. Date: may 36, 1998.

1442 Starks MA, et al. "The effects of phosphatidylserine on endocrine response to moderate intensity exercise." <u>J Int Soc Sports Nutr.</u> 2008, vol 5, p 11.

1443 Ralf Jager and Bokenkamp Kirk. "FORMULATION CONTAINING (LYSO-) PHOSPHATIDYLSERINE FOR THE PREVENTION AND TREATMENT OF STRESS STATES IN WARM BLOODED ANIMALS." Patent: US 2004/0234544 A1. Date Nov 25, 2004.

1444 Peale PK. "COMPOSITION OF PYRUVATE AND ANTICORTISOL COMPOUNDS AND METHOD FOR INCREASING PROTEIN CONCENTRATION IN A MAMMAL." Patent: 5,756,469. Date: may 36, 1998.

1445 Funfgeld EW, et al. "Double-blind study with phosphatidylserine (PS) in parkinsonian patients with senile dementia of Alzheimer's type (SDAT)." <u>Prog Clin Biol Res.</u> 1989, pp 1235-1246.

1446 McCleary EL. "COMPOSITION AND METHOD FOR TREATING IMPAIRED OR DETERIORATING NEUROLOGICAL FUNCTION." Patent: US 6,964,969 B2. Date: Nov 15, 2005.

1447 Funfgeld EW, et al. "Double-blind study with phosphatidylserine (PS) in parkinsonian patients with senile dementia of Alzheimer's type (SDAT)." <u>Prog Clin Biol Res.</u> 1989, pp 1235-1246.

1448 Jager R, et al. "Phospholipids and sports performance." <u>Journal of International Scoiety of Sports Nutrition.</u> 2007, vol 4, p 5.

1449 Murakami M, et al. "Change in Sensitivity to Lysophosphatidylserine of Mouse Bone Marrow-Derived Mast Cells during Cultivation with Fibroblasts." <u>Int Arch Allergy Immunol.</u> 1991, vol 96, PP 156-160.

[1450] Chauhan A and Chauhan V. "Oxidative stress in autism." Pathophysiology. 2006, vol 13(3), pp 171-181.